SECRETS OF
AROMATHERAPY

JENNIE HARDING

IVY PRESS

This edition published in the UK and North America in 2017 by
Ivy Press
An imprint of The Quarto Group
The Old Brewery, 6 Blundell Street
London N7 9BH, United Kingdom
T (0)20 7700 6700 **F** (0)20 7700 8066
www.QuartoKnows.com

First published in 2000

British Library Cataloguing-in-Publication Data
A catalogue record for this book is available from the British Library

ISBN: 978-1-78240-491-0

This book was conceived, designed and produced by
Ivy Press
58 West Street, Brighton BN1 2RA, United Kingdom

Art Director: Peter Bridgewater
Publisher: Sophie Collins
Editorial Director: Steve Luck
Designers: Kevin Knight, Jane Lanaway and Ginny Zeal
Editor: Rowan Davies
Picture Researcher: Liz Eddison
Photography: Guy Ryecart
Photography administration: Kay MacMullan
Illustrations: Sarah Young, Catherine McIntryre
and Michael Courtney
Three-dimensional models: Mark Jamieson
Assistant Editor: Jenny Campbell

Printed in China

10 9 8 7 6 5 4 3 2 1

Cover image: Getty/aromanta

MIX
Paper fro
responsible s
FSC® C008
www.fsc.org

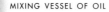

GERANIUM LEAF

HOW TO USE THIS BOOK To make this book a

useful introduction to aromatherapy, we have ordered it as follows: the first chapter, Aromatherapy, provides essential historical background; the second, Essential & Carrier Oils, gives in-depth information about the key essential oils and base products; and the third, Practical Aromatherapy, outlines self-massage techniques as well as describing what to expect at an aromatherapist's clinic. For information on a specific condition, turn to the second chapter, which categorizes oils by the bodily systems that they affect.

Important Notice

If you suffer from anxiety, depression, or any emotional problems that are seriously affecting your work, social life, or relationships you should seek the advice of your registered medical practitioner. It is also important to inform your doctor of any remedies or medications you are taking. If you ever feel that you might do harm to yourself or others you must seek immediate medical attention.

Aromatherapy should not be used as a replacement for conventional medical treatment.

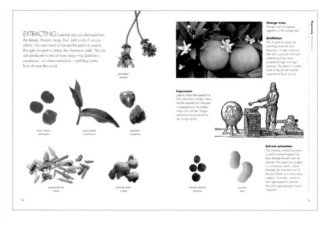

Background

The first chapter describes the historical origins and modern methods of aromatherapy.

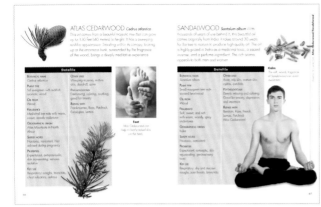

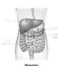

Oils

This chapter provides information on 30 key essential oils and 8 carrier oils.

Essential facts

The second chapter also analyzes bodily systems and the oils that affect them.

Essential Oils for Digestion

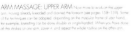

Digestion

Autotherapy can be of great assistance in treating digestion problems. We take a back of varying types and quality every day, yet are completely unaware of our digestive tract, busy extracting the nutrients and converting them for our use.

Tone up

We use often erratic in our eating patterns, and experience problems such as constipation because our digestion is sluggish. Essential oils can really help tone

up the digestion, to improve the rhythm of elimination, and to ease the underlying stress that can so often be an issue. Stress can quickly affect the digestive process, and abdominal massage, either self applied or by a professional, can quickly relieve muscular tension in the abdomen.

Eating habits

Poor eating habits can have a negative psychological impact on the system too. Eating meals when stressed, under pressure, angry, or while watching distractive images on television does not help to create relaxed digestion. Also, a sedentary lifestyle with little exercise does not stimulate enough rhythm in the large intestine to encourage regular elimination.

Try to achieve a balance between rest, relaxation, a healthy wholefood diet, regular exercise, and a positive attitude. Essential oils such as Black Pepper, Ginger, Peppermint, Lemongrass, Orange, or Roman Chamomile can all be used to help warm and soothe the abdominal area, and also have the effect of stimulating the appetite.

Safety

It is important to stress that essential oils are not swallowed to taken orally. The lining of the digestive tract is extremely sensitive, and would be damaged by this dosage. Essential oils can be used very effectively in a massage or in the bath to treat digestive problems.

There have been a number of cases of poisoning with large doses of essential oils that have been swallowed, sometimes by accident, so keep all essential oils out of the reach of children.

For children aged between three and ten, please halve any stated number of drops in a blend to the same amount of carrier product.

Key Essential Oil

Peppermint essential oil refreshes and eases the process of digestion.

Self-help

This final chapter gives you all the information you need to practice self-healing with aromatherapy.

ARM MASSAGE: UPPER ARM

Now move to work on the upper arm, moving slowly, kneaded and drained the forearm (see pages 158–159). Some of the techniques can be adapted, depending on the muscular frame of your friend, for example, kneading can be done double or single-handed. When you have done all the strokes on one arm, cover it and repeat the whole routine on the other arm.

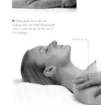

3 Now repeat the stroke all the way up the arm from the fingers to the shoulders, but this time apply more pressure on your upstroke and increase the speed to tone more digestion. The drains the whole arm.

4 Glide gently down the part, moving with one hand following the other to relax the arm at the end of the massage.

1 Supporting the arm with one hand at the level of the elbow, stroke firmly around the shoulder in a circular movement, five or five times.

2 Use one hand at both to knead the upper arm particularly the deltoid and biceps muscles. Spend a good few minutes on this.

Aromatherapy: A Gift from Nature

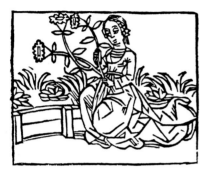

Aromatic
Throughout history, people have used plants for their aromatic properties.

When you walk past a rose bush, stop for a minute and inhale the cool sweet fragrance, pause and feel that sense of total well-being; you have just experienced aromatherapy. When you chop herbs in the kitchen and the pungent scents tingle in your nose and make your mouth water, there it is again. When you pass an Indian restaurant, notice how the warm spices arouse your senses. All of these fragrances are created by plants. They are contained in roots, leaves, fruits, flowers, and wood, and humankind has been drawn to use them in cooking, medicines, perfumes, and cosmetics for thousands of years.

Essential oils

These special fragrances are called "essential oils." They are extracted from their plant sources and used in aromatherapy, where they are directly applied to the body in order to improve relaxation and general well-being. Many of the oils can have a beneficial effect on particular symptoms in the body, helping to alleviate them. Aromatherapy also helps defuse mental and emotional stress, through the enjoyment of these beautiful, natural scents.

True aromatherapy

In the past 30 years, the use of these plant extracts for health and relaxation purposes has greatly increased. Essential oils can now be found in a whole host of widely available products, from toothpastes to shower gels, face creams, and body lotions. In every city, there are also many practitioners of aromatherapy massage who offer treatments. However, as aromatherapy becomes more popular, it is becoming more and more important for people to understand what true aromatherapy is all about, what essential oils are, and how they affect us. There are many products and treatments out there which are not all they would seem to be.

This book aims to guide you through all aspects of aromatherapy, giving you a real insight into essential oils so that you will be well-placed to use them on yourself, your family, and your friends, and experience true aromatherapy.

Key Essential Oil

Lavender is often one of the first essential oils used in aromatherapy.

AROMATHERAPY

Aromatherapy uses "aromas," essential oils from plants, as a "therapy," a way of improving a person's health and well-being. Applying essential oils with massage, or in baths, inhalations, and vaporizers can have significantly positive effects on a person's mood, as well as easing physical aches and pains. Working with aromatherapy requires a careful choice and application of essential oils, in the appropriate carrier product. Therefore, you need to know the oils well, and have a good understanding of when and how to apply them to achieve maximum benefits to your health. Aromatherapy is a beautiful art, pleasing to the senses and a joy to receive. It is also a natural way of enhancing and maintaining good health and a positive mental attitude.

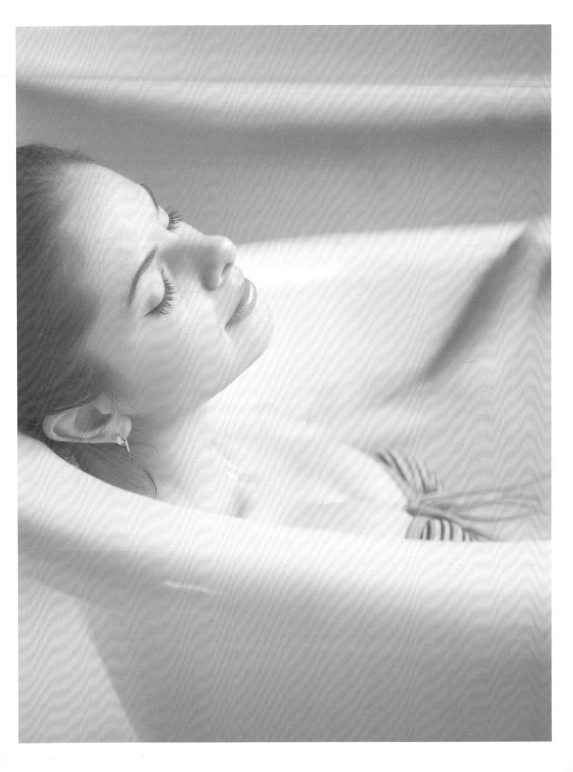

Origins of Aromatherapy

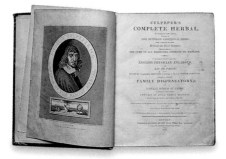

Herbal
*Nicholas Culpeper published
a famous herbal in 1653, which
described the properties of herbs.*

Aromatherapy as it is practiced today has its roots in antiquity, when aromatic herbs and essences were used as cosmetics, medicines, perfumes, and incense.

Aromatic history

In Ancient Egypt, herbs were steeped in fat and left in the sun. The heat drew out the aroma, which merged into the oily base to create ointments and solid perfumes. The practice of embalming the bodies of dead Pharaohs involved packing aromatic gums, spices, and woods into body cavities. In the tomb of Tutankhamen, alabaster jars were found containing ointments that could still be analyzed thousands of years later, and were found to contain gums such as frankincense and myrrh, which, along with cedarwood and other spices, were used in embalming.

The Ancient Greek physician Hippocrates, born about 460 BCE, advised that scented herbs should be burned over his patients. Other physicians created herbal remedies such as "megaleion," which contained myrrh and cinnamon and could be used as a wound-healing treatment as well as a fragrance.

Distillation

The great Arab scholar Avicenna (980–1037 CE) is credited with rediscovering techniques of distillation, which he applied to the rose, obtaining aromatic waters and essential oil. Artifacts found in Iraq and Pakistan suggest that distillation may have been in use several thousand years ago. Distillation continued to be used during the Middle Ages and into the 16th and 17th centuries. At this time, herbals, small books describing the process of extraction and descriptions of the properties of herbs, were printed.

Herbal treatments and essential oils were the medicine of the people, as described by Nicholas Culpeper in his famous herbal of 1653. Later in that century when bubonic plague raged through Europe, physicians wore masks stuffed with herbs and spices to protect them from infection. In the 18th century, in apothecary shops in London, it was possible to buy herbal remedies containing essential oils. However, with the growth of interest in synthetic, so called "pure," drugs during the 19th century, essential oils and herbs fell largely into disuse in the West, but the 20th century saw a revival of interest in herbs and essential oils.

Key Essential Oil

The fragrance of **Frankincense** connects us to the history of aromatherapy.

EXTRACTING

Essential oils are obtained from the leaves, flowers, twigs, fruit, and roots of various plants. Growers need to harvest the plant at exactly the right moment to obtain the maximum yield. The oils are produced in one of three ways—by distillation, expression, or solvent extraction—and they come from all over the world.

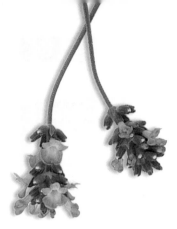

LAVENDER
FRANCE

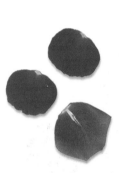

ROSE PETALS
BULGARIA

EUCALYPTUS
AUSTRALIA

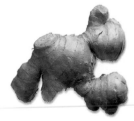

BENZOIN
SUMATRA

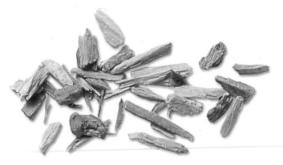

SANDALWOOD
INDIA

GINGER ROOT
CHINA

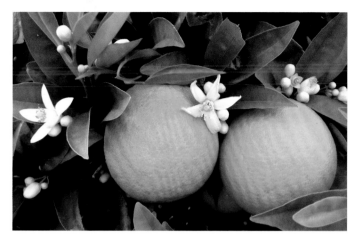

Orange trees
Flowers and fruit appear together on the orange tree.

Distillation
This is used for many oils, including Lavender and Rosemary. A steel container (the still) is packed with plant material and has steam pumped through it at high pressure. The steam is cooled back to liquid form and the essential oil floats on top.

Expression
Used to obtain the essential oil from citrus fruits, it simply means that the essential oil in the peel is squeezed out. Nowadays, many citrus oils like Orange and Lemon are produced by the juicing industry.

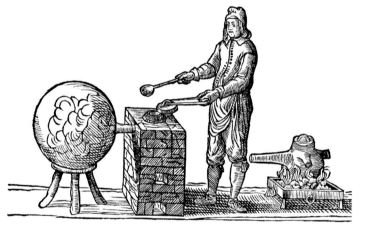

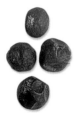

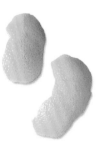

JUNIPER BERRIES
CROATIA

LEMON
ITALY

Solvent extraction
This complex chemical process is used to extract fragrant oils from delicate flowers such as jasmine. The petals are soaked in a chemical solvent, which dissolves the aromatics out of the plant fibers as a sticky mass called a "concrete," which is then reprocessed to remove fats and waxes giving a liquid "absolute."

Modern Aromatherapy

The term "aromatherapy" was first used by René-Maurice Gattefossé, a French perfume chemist who used neat lavender oil in a laboratory accident to heal a burn on his hand. He then used essential oils to treat hospitalized soldiers during World War I. In the late 1920s and 30s he continued to study essential oils as potential healing agents. Another French doctor, Jean Valnet, used essential oils as treatments for war wounds in the Indo-China war of 1948–1959; he went on to become a father of aromatherapy, producing a classic text, *Aromatherapie*, in 1964, where he called essential oils the potential "stars of medicine." Valnet's work was studied in turn by Marguerite Maury, who created aromatherapy as it tends to be practiced today, with the emphasis on an individual prescription of essential oils to match a person's psychological state as well as their physical condition. Maury also proposed the notion of massage as a means of administering the oils.

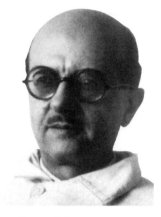

Essential treatment
René-Maurice Gattefossé, a French perfume chemist, the "father" of modern aromatherapy.

Robert Tisserand

The first book in English, *The Art of Aromatherapy*, was published by Robert Tisserand in 1975. It brought together historical information on essential oils and a detailed methodology for their use, and has been translated into several languages. Tisserand is a major figure in aromatherapy around the world. His work now includes the extensive text *Essential Oil Safety*, a key manual for therapists and practitioners.

Essential oils rediscovered

Aromatherapy is still evolving. The practice of aromatherapy has many aspects: on the one hand it can be a fragrant massage, but on the other it plays an ever more vital role in today's stressed and fast-moving world. Essential oils are increasingly being used in hospitals, residential homes for seniors, schools, on aircraft, and in the workplace. The practice of vaporizing oils is even being called "environmental fragrancing" and is helping to beat "sick building" syndrome. Modern buildings with central heating and air conditioning systems are constantly recycling germs into the air, spreading infection. Essential oils like Tea Tree can help disinfect the environment and improve the air quality. The recent rediscovery of essential oils is truly an aromatic revolution.

Key Essential Oil

Tea Tree is invaluable as an antiseptic and wound-healer.

Smooth as a peach

The kernel of the peach yields a light textured massage oil.

OILS & CARRIERS

An essential oil is a very fragrant liquid that evaporates quickly in warm temperatures. It is extremely concentrated—approximately 0.75 ton (760 kilograms) of lavender plant is needed to produce approximately 3½ pints (2 liters) of lavender oil.

A carrier oil is a vegetable oil that is used to dilute the essential oils and make them safe for use in massage. A blend of essential oils diluted in a vegetable oil, like sweet almond or grapeseed, is gentle on the skin. Base lotions and creams are also available. These carrier products are suited to specific uses, and are especially good for the skin.

The right measure

Measuring spoons can be obtained from a pharmacy.

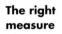

1 *Use a funnel to pour larger amounts of carrier oil into your mixing bottle.*

2 *Drops of pure essential oil can be accurately added to the carrier oil due to the special stopper in the neck of the essential oil bottle.*

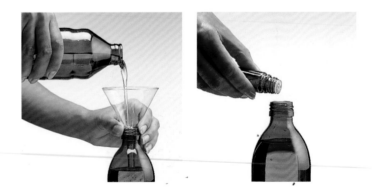

Essential Oils Guidelines

Here are guidelines to help you choose the right dose of essential oils for the blend you want to make.

10 drops total of essential oils in 20ml/4 teaspoons of carrier oil is a 2.5% dilution

This is safe for normal adult skin.
No sensitivities or allergies to perfume.

5 drops total of essential oils in 20ml/4 teaspoons of carrier oil is a 1% dilution

This is safe for adults with sensitive skin, or children aged 3–10 years; it can also be used to make a massage blend to apply during pregnancy—but only after the 12th week.
For the first 3 months of pregnancy, no essential oils should be used in massage (see page 20).

You can see that to make a 1% dilution, you divide the number of drops in a 2.5% dilution by half. Further on in this book, we give you many different ideas for blends to try—these are at 2.5%. If you have sensitive skin, you should always divide the number of drops in half in the same amount of carrier oil.

Safety

The most common dilution shown in this book is for **normal skin only**. Anyone with sensitive skin must use **half the stated dose** of drops in the same amount of carrier base.

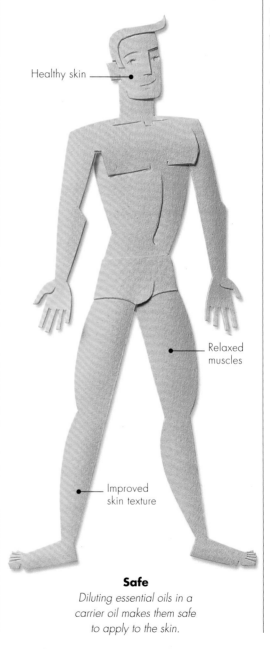

Healthy skin

Relaxed muscles

Improved skin texture

Safe
Diluting essential oils in a carrier oil makes them safe to apply to the skin.

Therapeutic Guidelines

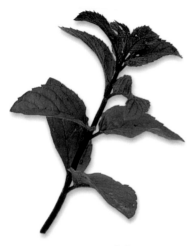

Be careful
Although essential oils are natural substances they must be used carefully.

There are some basic rules that need to be observed in order to use essential oils safely. The essential oils featured in this book have been chosen because they have very few safety issues, and if you follow the instructions given you are very unlikely to experience any problems. However, the following pieces of general information should be taken into consideration at all times. If you are unsure about using essential oils you should consult a qualified therapist.

General safety

Do not swallow essential oils; they can irritate the digestive tract, and in large doses may do internal damage. Do not use them neat on the skin; exceptions to this rule are Lavender and Tea Tree oils, which can be used for first-aid purposes. Keep all essential oils out of the reach of children. Observe the shelf life of your essential oils (see pages 28–29). If oils are past their shelf life they are more likely to cause irritation.

Essential oils should be avoided for the first three months of pregnancy, and then only a 1 percent dilution should be used for massage. It is recommended that, during pregnancy, you use only gentle oils like Mandarin, Orange, Palmarosa, or Neroli.

The essential oils of Peppermint or Rosemary are not recommended for those with high blood pressure.

Skin safety

If you have highly sensitive skin you need to patch test all essential oils before you use them (see pages 22–23). If you find an essential oil causes a red rash, wash the area with mild soap and apply plain Sweet Almond carrier oil to soothe the skin.

All the citrus oils—Bergamot, Lemon, Orange, and Mandarin—are potentially phototoxic, causing irregular pigmentation in ultraviolet (UV) light. Therefore, if you have used a blend containing a citrus oil stay out of strong UV light, such as sunlight or a sunbed, for 12 hours after application.

Child safety

Essential oils should not be massaged into the skin of newborns or babies up to 12 months old. Just use a plain carrier oil such as Apricot Kernel oil or Jojoba to nourish the skin. After that time, 1 drop of either Lavender or Roman Chamomile essential oil in 4 teaspoons (20 milliliters) of carrier oil makes a pleasant daily massage blend.

Key Essential Oil

Palmarosa is very gentle on the skin and in general use.

Adverse reactions

Applying a tiny amount of a blend under a bandage is a test for irritation.

TESTING AN OIL

There are two methods you can use to test your reactions to particular essential oils. The first test helps you discover the effects of different essential oils on your mood and feelings; you may feel uplifted, cheered, or refreshed by the fragrances. The second test is a patch test to see if your skin reacts to essential oils. You should be careful to do a patch test if you know that you have sensitive skin.

1 *Sit comfortably in a chair in a room where you will not be disturbed. Take a few breaths and relax.*

2 *In 2 teaspoons (10 milliliters) of grapeseed oil add 2 drops of a chosen essential oil. Stir gently into the carrier.*

3 *Apply a small amount of this blend to your wrists, rub in well, wait for a moment to allow the fragrance to develop on your skin.*

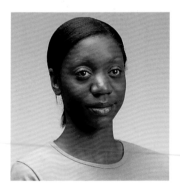

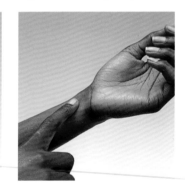

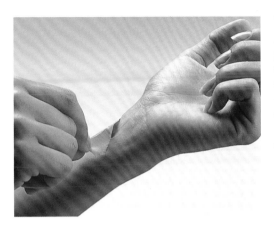

The skin patch test

In 2 teaspoons (10 milliliters) of grapeseed oil add 4 drops of your chosen essential oil. Apply a small amount of blend on the inside of your wrist or elbow crease, and cover with a bandage. Leave for 12 hours and remove. If there is no redness, go ahead and use the oil.

5 *After your smell test, rub a little arrowroot powder on the area to reduce the intensity of the fragrance.*

4 *Now smell your wrists, noticing how you react to the fragrance— how does it affect your mood, do you notice any physical effects?*

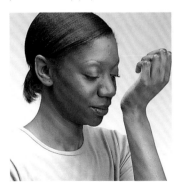

Proportions & Synergy

Olfactory bulb and pathway to brain center

Smell receptor cells

Fast acting
The sense of smell reacts in the brain in less than 2 seconds.

When you are learning about aromatherapy it is important to know the oils individually, in terms of their fragrance, properties, and uses. However, the second important dimension involves knowing how to blend several oils together in a balanced way.

Fragrance notes

In the 19th century, a Frenchman called George Piesse came up with the idea of classifying fragrances in terms of musical notes. Although much of his philosophy is no longer used, the notion of top, middle, and base notes still persists in perfumery, and the same principle can apply in aromatherapy. However, there are no rigid classifications of essential oils as fragrance notes; they tend to fall into one main category, though they may have other, more subtle characteristics.

If you are blending a total of 10 drops of a combination of essential oils in 4 teaspoons (20 milliliters) of carrier oil, this is how the notes work. The top notes (4–5 drops) evaporate most quickly and give a fresh light note. These are usually the citrus oils such as Mandarin or Lemon, or fresh oils such as Rosemary. The middle notes (3–4 drops) are the heart of the blend. Examples of these are Lavender, Geranium, and Petitgrain. The base notes (1–2 drops) are the deep and sometimes musky notes that evaporate slowly and linger the longest, for example Patchouli, Vetiver, and Jasmine. The blends suggested in this book generally follow this pattern.

Synergy

Synergy describes the process of essential oils working together therapeutically. You need to know the properties of each essential oil individually to know what to blend together for the best effect. If you want a pain-relieving blend, then it helps to use three painkilling oils rather than just one. However, if you want a blend for pain relief and stress, you may choose two painkillers and another oil to uplift mental anxiety. A simple blend of two essential oils is pleasant to use. Three essential oils may be a well-balanced fragrance, which also works synergistically, on body and mind. This is the combination most often used for holistic aromatherapy massage treatment. You will find that blends of two or three oils are featured regularly throughout this book.

Key Essential Oil

Rose essential oil is one of the most complex fragrances in aromatherapy.

ACTIVE METHODS OF USE

There are a number of methods you can use to infuse your body with essential oils and promote an overall sense of well-being. Massage is most often used, compresses and baths can be easily prepared at home, and inhalation is great for attacking colds and the flu.

Blends

Pour a small amount of blend into your hand to start massaging.

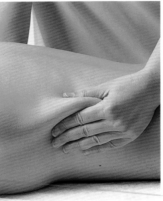

Massage

A massage works a blend of essential oils and carrier oil into the skin. There are three basic techniques that are most often used. Effleurage describes a stroking motion that warms the skin, kneading picks up the muscle and squeezes it, while pressure uses small circular strokes. For more information on massage methods refer to chapter 3.

1 *Effleurage means using the whole of the palm of your hand in contact with the skin, stroking to warm the muscles and spread the blend.*

2 *Kneading involves picking up skin and muscle and squeezing it out, like making bread dough. This eases out the tension.*

3 *Pressures are small circular movements performed with the thumb on areas that are knotted or tight. Apply pressure for 20 seconds, then release and stroke the area.*

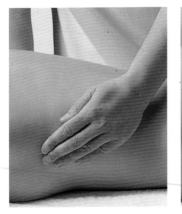

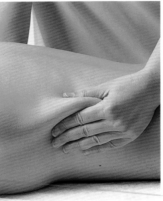

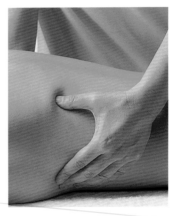

Pamper yourself
Aromatherapy is a way to relax at the end of the day.

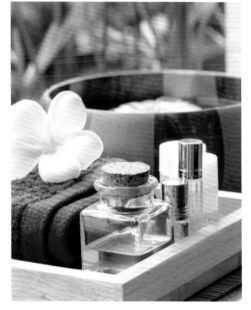

To use aromatherapy in the bath

 First fill it to a comfortable temperature. Sprinkle a total of 6 drops of essential oil onto the surface and agitate the water. Alternatively, dilute the oil in 6 teaspoons (30 milliliters) of whole milk and add this to the bath to soften the water. Soak for 20 minutes.

Footbath

 In a large bowl of warm water add 4–5 drops of essential oil. Soak the feet for 20 minutes.

Compresses

 Hot compresses will draw out poison—a skin infection, for example—and cold compresses will ease pain and inflammation, such as a sprained ankle.

To make a compress, fill a bowl with hot or cold water and add 2 to 3 drops of one essential oil. Place a thin cloth over the surface of the water to soak up the essential oil. Wring out the cloth and apply it to the appropriate area for 15 to 20 minutes.

Inhalation of essential oils

 This is particularly effective for soothing the symptoms of colds or the flu. Fill a large bowl with near-boiling water. Add 3 drops each of useful oils such as Tea Tree and Eucalyptus. Remove glasses or contact lenses, then, with a towel over your head, lean over the bowl and breathe in the vapors for 15 minutes.

Instant treatment
Preparing an inhalation requires only simple equipment.

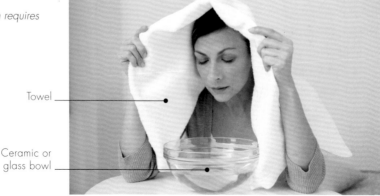

Towel

Ceramic or glass bowl

Buying & Storing Essential Oils

When buying essential oils there are a few things to first consider. Oils are best purchased in dark glass bottles protecting them from ultraviolet (UV) light, which speeds up their deterioration. All bottles should have a tight-fitting stopper that dispenses the oil one drop at a time. This not only helps when making blends, but also presents minimum risk of swallowing if the bottle accidentally comes into contact with a child's mouth. Do not buy essential oils in open-necked bottles because of increased risk of accidental ingestion of large quantities of oil.

Both the Latin name as well as the common English name of the oil should appear on the label. There are several different Lavender and Eucalyptus varieties available, so you need to be sure of exactly what you are buying. A good supplier will be willing and able to provide all the necessary information about the oil, its active constituents, geographical origin, and freshness.

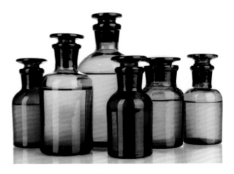

Storage
Dark glass bottles with stoppers are recommended, because light can affect the contents.

Storing

Storing essential oils also requires some forethought. Essential oils are one hundred percent natural extracts from plants. Because they are from living organisms they do have a shelf life, and will eventually deteriorate, losing their fragrance or becoming cloudy or sticky in the bottle. Key considerations when storing oils, therefore, are light, temperature, and moisture. Your oils are best stored in the refrigerator for the maximum shelf life; if this is problematic because of children, then try to find a cool, dark, dry place. If you do keep them in the refrigerator, put them in an airtight container to keep them separate from foods, particularly dairy products. If kept in this way, the shelf life of citrus oils such as Lemon, Orange, Mandarin, or Bergamot should be one year, while all other oils should last two years. If the oils are not refrigerated, then citrus oils will stay usable for six months; all other oils will keep for one year. It is a good idea to write the date on the label when you open the bottle to remind you of how long you should store it.

You are recommended to use essential oils that are as fresh as possible. Once they have passed their shelf life they can deteriorate and can cause skin reactions.

Key Essential Oil

Bergamot, like all citrus oils, has a shorter shelf life (6–12 months).

29

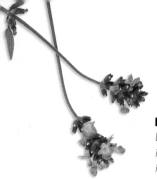

Relaxing
*Using 4–6 drops of Lavender
in a vaporizer can help you relax
into sleep.*

PASSIVE METHODS OF USE Passive methods of use are ways
of spreading the fragrance of essential oils into a room so that the aromas can be
enjoyed immediately; the essential oils are inhaled but do not come into direct contact
with the body. Vaporizers in particular are useful in the bedroom.

Dish for water and
essential oils

Vaporizers
*These are ceramic units that are either electrical or
require a small candle. Sprinkle 4 to 6 drops of
essential oils into the unit and, as it heats up, the
oils fragrance the room.*

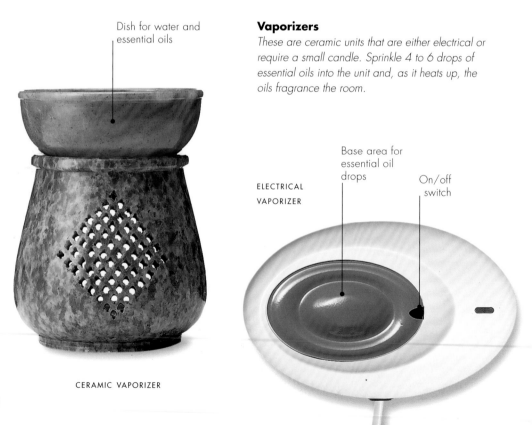

Base area for
essential oil
drops

On/off
switch

ELECTRICAL
VAPORIZER

CERAMIC VAPORIZER

Refreshing

Essential oil of Rosemary is pungent and fresh.

Mist sprays

These help to humidify a room, as well as freshen the air. Add 15 drops in total of two essential oils to 7 fluid ounces (200 milliliters) of water. Shake and spray the liquid into the air.

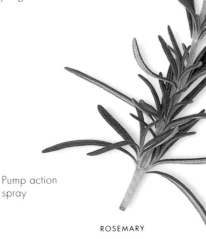

Pump action spray

ROSEMARY

Candles

Alternatively, candles containing essential oils in the wax can also be used. The oils evaporate as the candle burns, although their effect is more pleasing than therapeutic.

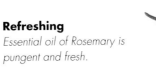

Water with essential oils

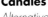

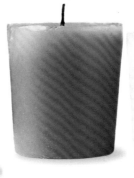

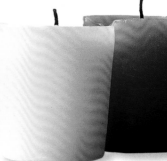

Q&A

QUESTIONS & ANSWERS

As a beginner, you will probably have a lot of questions about the whole field of aromatherapy. Here are some common questions about aromatherapy and essential oils that people often ask. If the answers here don't quite meet your needs, bear in mind that it is always a good idea to discuss any issues that concern you with a qualified practitioner.

Q Are essential oils dangerous?

A *Only if they are swallowed in large amounts. In aromatherapy we stress that the oils should never be taken internally. Used diluted on the skin, in the bath, inhaled, or vaporized they are very beneficial.*

Q Can you use too much essential oil?

A *Again, they can harm you if you swallow large amounts of them. If you bathe with them, inhale occasionally for colds or the flu, and have a regular massage treatment you will feel them enhance your energy and well-being.*

Q Can you use essential oils on babies?

A *Essential oils should not be massaged into the skin of newborns or babies up to 12 months old. Just use a plain carrier oil to nourish the skin. See page 21 for when it is safe to begin using essential oils in a daily massage blend.*

Q Do I need to use water in my vaporizer?

A It depends on the design. Some have deep bowls where water can be used, others are very shallow, and in that case the oil can be used without water.

Q How often should I have aromatherapy treatment?

A It depends on why you are having treatment. If you have a straightforward physical problem, such as stiff shoulders, four or five weekly sessions should see some improvement. If you have a chronic problem, like arthritis, you may need a few months of treatment before you begin to feel better. Your therapist should tell you how many sessions you may need.

Q Do the oils really get into the body?

A Yes. Through massage and baths, essential oils work their way through the skin and into the bloodstream. From vaporizing or inhalation, aromatic molecules reach the lungs.

Q Can I use oils at work to stop germs from spreading?

A Yes. Try using an electrical vaporizer close to your workstation, with 3 drops of Tea Tree and 3 drops of Lemon. Or you could put a few drops of essential oil on a tissue and sniff it periodically.

Q I don't like Lavender. What else can relax me?

A Try Rosewood, Sandalwood, or Ylang Ylang as alternatives.

Q Is aromatherapy only for women?

A No—the variety of essential oils used includes many fragrances that are appealing to men; including Patchouli, Rosemary, and Cypress.

ESSENTIAL
& CARRIER OILS

This section of the book features 30 key essential oils that form a comprehensive kit for home use. Each oil has its own factfile that gives important information on its origin, its physical and psychological uses, as well as safety advice and ideas for blending. The oils are organized into groups linked to particular problem areas, with the key uses for each oil emphasized, enabling you to make appropriate choices when working on yourself, family, and friends. We then move on to examine 8 carrier oils in the same format. Discover for yourself the gentle healing qualities of essential oils. They are fun to collect and interesting to learn about as well as practical in use. By inhaling these beautiful natural fragrances and working them into the skin you will experience the magic of aromatherapy.

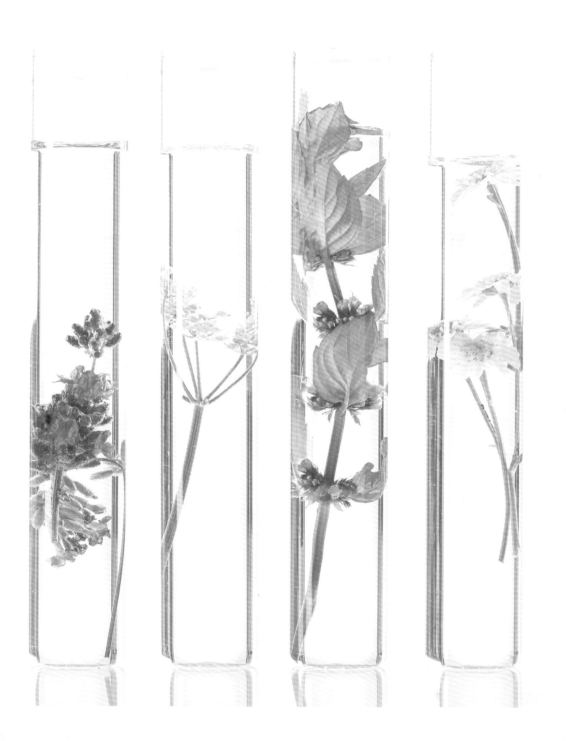

Essential Oils for the Skin & Hair

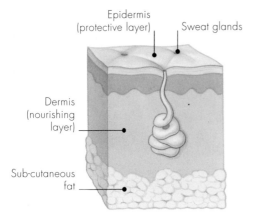

Epidermis (protective layer)

Sweat glands

Dermis (nourishing layer)

Sub-cutaneous fat

Skin

The skin is made up of three distinct layers.

Using aromatherapy to help skin problems is one of the best ways to observe what the oils are actually doing. As patches of redness fade, blemishes heal, inflammation is reduced, and the skin responds to the toning properties of essential oils, the result is a much clearer, more even complexion, which is soft to the touch.

To understand how aromatherapy can help skin problems, it helps to know about the structure of the skin (see diagram).

Skin care

Essential oils can rejuvenate and rebuild the upper skin layer by removing old cells and stimulating new growth. They can also improve local circulation and muscle tone, encourage the removal of waste products, reduce inflammation, clear infection, and minimize scarring.

Carrier oils

Essential oils need to be blended in the correct type of carrier product, depending on the problem. Vegetable oils, lotions, or creams may be appropriate. Vegetable oils are good all-round conditioners. Base lotion is a cooling carrier product because of its higher water content and so is good for areas of redness or inflammation. Base cream is a skin lubricating carrier and is excellent for targeting damaged skin. Essential oils can be absorbed much more easily through damaged skin so it is important that you follow the blends and methods suggested.

Hair care

Your hair is alive only at the root, and dead once it is outside the skin layer. It is made up of a protein called keratin, and is normally lubricated by special glands in the skin that secrete natural oils along the shaft. Use of bleaches, harsh shampoos, and hair processing products can dry out the scalp as well as strip the hair of its natural oils. Aromatherapy scalp massages help to feed the roots of the hair, which in turn encourages healthy hair growth. Blends of essential oils can also smooth the texture of the hair, as well as giving it a wonderful fragrance. See page 41 for special aromatherapy treatments to really pamper and nourish your hair and achieve the most beautiful results.

Key Essential Oil

Roman Chamomile is soothing to the outer skin layers and is often used as an anti-inflammatory.

FRANKINCENSE *Boswellia carterii*

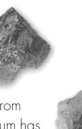

Frankincense is famous for being one of the gifts brought by the wise men to the infant Christ at His birth. The name stems from old French and means "true incense." Historically, frankincense gum has been burned in temples, churches, and places of worship for millennia. Vaporized, frankincense creates a beautifully calm atmosphere, which helps set the scene for meditation, quiet time, or yoga practice.

Datafile

BOTANICAL NAME
Boswella carterii

PLANT TYPE
Small tree with spiky leaves and pinkish flowers. The gum is formed in the bark

OIL FROM
Gum

FRAGRANCE
Sharp, fresh top note, becoming warmer. Richer and more resiny later

GEOGRAPHICAL ORIGIN
Somalia, Ethiopia

SAFETY NOTES
Nontoxic, nonirritant

PROPERTIES
Skin reviving, toning and soothing, expectorant, immune stimulant

KEY USE
Skin care: for dry and mature skin, acne, scar tissue, eczema

OTHER USES
Asthma, bronchitis, colds, the flu

PSYCHOLOGICALLY
Use for anxiety and nervous tension. It is calming and spiritually uplifting

BLENDS WITH
Grapefruit, Orange, Lemon, Lavender, Sandalwood, Patchouli, Rose

Incense
Frankincense was one of the gifts given to the infant Jesus.

ROMAN CHAMOMILE *Anthemis nobilis* This is a very gentle oil,

highly valued as a remedy for children's upsets, whether physical or emotional, as well as a fine skin care ingredient. It has more than two thousand years of use behind it in Western herbal medicine. In the garden, it will keep other plants healthy and pest-free.

Datafile

BOTANICAL NAME
Anthemis nobilis

PLANT TYPE
Small perennial plant with a strong, apple-like odor and white daisy flowers

OIL FROM
Flowering tops

FRAGRANCE
Sweet, fruity and soft, slightly herbaceous

GEOGRAPHICAL ORIGIN
United Kingdom

SAFETY NOTES
Nontoxic, nonirritant

PROPERTIES
Soothing, anti-inflammatory, antispasmodic, nerve sedative

KEY USE
Skin care: burns, cuts, allergies, eczema, inflammation, rashes

OTHER USES
Muscular aches and pains, inflamed joints, indigestion

PSYCHOLOGICALLY
Very calming to the nerves. Good for headache, migraines, and stress

BLENDS WITH
Lavender, Bergamot, Neroli, Sandalwood, Peppermint, Palmarosa

Gentle
Roman Chamomile is soothing on the skin.

Roman Chamomile flowers

The leaves have an apple-like aroma

Skincare Conditions & Treatments

The numbers next to the oils refer to the number of drops to be used. Halve the number of drops used for children between three and ten years old.

CONDITION	OILS	METHOD
Acne: red, pus-filled pimples with yellow heads	4 Tea Tree 3 Sandalwood 3 Lavender	These essential oils in 4 teaspoons (20 milliliters) of base lotion. Apply twice daily
Allergies: raised, red, itching areas. If severe seek medical help	2 Roman Chamomile	Apply a cold compress to the area for 20 minutes
Athlete's foot: fungal infection between the toes	4 Tea Tree 3 Lavender	These essential oils in a warm footbath. Soak the feet for 20 minutes twice daily
Boils: infected, swollen lumps under the skin. If severe, seek medical help	3 Bergamot 3 Lavender	Apply a hot compress to the area twice daily
Bruises: injury under the skin, pain, swelling, blue marking	2 Peppermint 3 Roman Chamomile	Apply an ice-cold compress to the area for 20 minutes
Cracked skin: damage to heels, for example	4 Frankincense 6 Lavender	These essential oils in 4 teaspoons (20 grams) of base cream or 4 teaspoons (20 milliliters) of sweet almond oil. Apply twice daily
Chilblains: reddish-blue swellings often on toes, due to poor circulation	4 Black Pepper 3 Ginger	These essential oils in a comfortably hot footbath. Soak the feet for 20 minutes. Then massage the feet with these oils repeated in 2 teaspoons (10 milliliters) of sweet almond oil

Hair Care Treatment

An aromatherapy hair pack treatment can help to take care of the scalp and hair.

Take 4 teaspoons (20 milliliters) of sweet almond oil, and add the appropriate blend of essential oils as listed below. Massage the blend into dry hair. Cover the head with a towel for 20 minutes. Then apply shampoo straight into the hair and rinse as normal. Do this once a week for a month.

Suggested Blends for Specific Hair Types

The numbers next to the oils refer to the number of drops to be used.

Dry hair:	3 Rose, 7 Sandalwood
Oily hair:	4 Juniper, 6 Petitgrain
Dull hair:	4 Patchouli, 6 Palmarosa
Normal hair:	4 Frankincense, 6 Orange
Dandruff:	4 Tea Tree, 6 Geranium
Hair loss:	5 Rosemary, 5 Ginger

Key Essential Oil

Patchouli is an excellent all-round skin and hair tonic, and can also help aid digestion.

LAVENDER *Lavandula angustifolia*

The lavender plant was first introduced to Great Britain by the Romans and it has since enjoyed popularity throughout history as a cottage garden flower. The south of France, mainly Provence, produces a great deal of the oil, and it is also distilled from the fields of Norfolk in the United Kingdom. Lavender water is a by-product of distillation and can be used as a toner for combination or dry skin.

Datafile

BOTANICAL NAME
Lavandula angustifolia

PLANT TYPE
Evergreen shrub up to 3 feet (1 meter) tall, with light green narrow leaves and violet blue flowers on long stalks

OIL FROM
Flowering tops

FRAGRANCE
Fruity and fresh top note, floral and woody undertones

GEOGRAPHICAL ORIGIN
France

SAFETY NOTES
Nontoxic, nonirritant

PROPERTIES
Painkilling, antiseptic, skin rejuvenating, antispasmodic, nerve sedative

KEY USE
Skin care: can be used neat on skin for cuts, burns, and first aid. Also tones and soothes the skin, heals acne and blemishes

OTHER USES
Muscular aches, indigestion, stomachaches, headaches, migraines, irritated or mucous coughs

PSYCHOLOGICALLY
One of the most calming oils, excellent for insomnia and anxiety

BLENDS WITH
Neroli, Sandalwood, Lemon, Peppermint

Scented

Lavender sachets can be used to perfume linen.

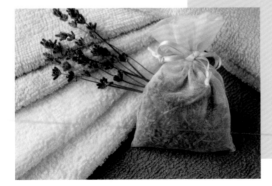

PATCHOULI *Pogostemon cablin*

In Victorian and Edwardian times there was a fashion for shawls from India scented with patchouli; the oil was used to preserve the cloth by acting as an insect repellent. The fragrance of the oil is very exotic, and it is extensively used in perfumery. It appeals to both men and women, with a reputation as an aphrodisiac. The dried, powdered leaves give incense a deep earthy fragrance.

Datafile

BOTANICAL NAME
Pogostemon cablin

PLANT TYPE
Perennial, bushy herb up to 3 feet (1 meter) in height with large, velvety leaves smelling strongly of the oil

OIL FROM
Leaves

FRAGRANCE
Rich, earthy, warming, and sweet

GEOGRAPHICAL ORIGIN
India, Indonesia

SAFETY NOTES
Nontoxic, nonirritant

PROPERTIES
Anti-inflammatory, skin rejuvenating, digestive tonic, nerve sedative

KEY USE
Skin care: acne, eczema, sore, chapped, or mature skin, scalp tonic

OTHER USES
Indigestion, stomachaches, digestive migraines

PSYCHOLOGICALLY
Calming, grounding, helps nervous exhaustion. Also considered to be an aphrodisiac

BLENDS WITH
Sandalwood, Frankincense, Lemon, Orange, Lavender

Leaves
Patchouli leaves are velvety in texture and strongly aromatic.

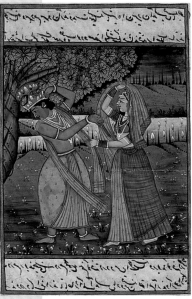

Oils for Skin & Hair • 2

Skincare Conditions & Treatments

The numbers next to the oils refer to the number of drops to be used. Halve the number of drops used for children between three and ten years old.

CONDITION	OILS	METHOD
Cold sores (herpes simplex), blisters, and scabs	2 Tea Tree	Place essential oil drops on a cotton swab and apply neat, twice daily
Cuts and bruises	5 Lavender 5 Tea Tree	These essential oils in 4 teaspoons (20 milliliters) base lotion for instant first aid. Apply twice daily, cover with a bandage
Eczema/dermatitis: patches of cracked skin in creases or folds, between the fingers, for example	2 Rose 8 Roman Chamomile	These essential oils in 4 teaspoons (20 milliliters) of base lotion. Apply twice daily
Psoriasis: large areas of tender skin with tiny white flakes peeling off; the epidermis is thin	3 Neroli 7 Frankincense	These essential oils in 4 teaspoons (20 grams) of base cream. Apply to the affected area twice daily
Sunburn	4 Roman Chamomile 6 Lavender	These essential oils in 4 teaspoons (20 milliliters) of base lotion. Apply as necessary
Rashes: urticaria (nettle rash), heat bumps. If rash persists seek medical help	2 Palmarosa 3 Roman Chamomile	Apply a cold compress to the affected area for 20 minutes
Congested/dull skin: due to poor diet or effects of central heating	4 Frankincense 6 Lemon	These essential oils in 4 teaspoons (20 milliliters) of Jojoba oil. Massage half a teaspoonful into the affected area daily

Insect Repellents & Bite Treatments

There are a few very useful oils to know about when on vacation, or if you live in a hot climate. Aromatherapy blends can be effectively used to help keep away mosquitoes.

Mix 4 drops Patchouli and 6 drops Lavender, or 3 drops Lemongrass and 7 drops Atlas Cedarwood in 4 teaspoons (20 milliliters) of sweet almond oil. Apply to clean skin in the evenings when the mosquitoes are active. In a vaporizer at night, try 3 drops Lemongrass and 3 drops Lavender to keep the insects at bay.

If you are bitten, apply 2 drops of neat Tea Tree on a cotton swab to the bite immediately. Tea Tree is effective against insect venom, fights infection, and should be used three times a day.

Key Essential Oil

Lemongrass is fragrant, zesty smelling, and can be used as a good insect repellent.

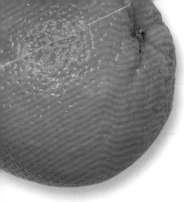

ORANGE *Citrus sinensis*

The Latin name means Chinese orange, and the tree was originally native to China. The fruit peel is crushed to remove the oil, and its sweet, pleasant fragrance makes it very popular in the perfumery, cosmetic, and flavoring industries. It is a gentle oil useful as a digestive tonic, especially for children. Adults will find it mouth-wateringly fresh as well.

Datafile

BOTANICAL NAME
Citrus sinensis

PLANT TYPE
Small evergreen tree yielding edible oranges

OIL FROM
Fruit peel

FRAGRANCE
Sweet, fresh, fruity

GEOGRAPHICAL ORIGIN
United States, Brazil

SAFETY NOTES
Nontoxic, nonirritant. Phototoxic. Do not expose skin to ultraviolet (UV) light for 12 hours after the application of a blend

PROPERTIES
Antiseptic, skin tonic, digestive tonic, nervous sedative

KEY USE
Skin care: for oily and combination skins, dull complexions, teenage acne

OTHER USES
Indigestion, constipation, sluggish digestion

PSYCHOLOGICALLY
A wonderful antidepressant oil, gentle and sweet, stress-relieving

BLENDS WITH
Petitgrain, Neroli, Lavender, Geranium, Peppermint

Digestion
Orange is a particular favorite with children. It helps with digestion.

NEROLI *Citrus aurantium* var. *amara* Neroli

(orange blossom) is a beautiful floral oil, although, because of the high numbers of flowers required to produce only a small amount, it is also costly. Orange flowers were traditionally used in bridal bouquets because the soft, calming fragrance was said to ease the bride's nerves.

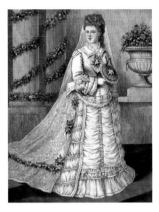

Datafile

BOTANICAL NAME
Citrus aurantium var. *amara*

PLANT TYPE
Evergreen tree up to 33 feet (10 meters) in height, with shiny dark green leaves and fragrant white flowers

OIL FROM
Flowers

FRAGRANCE
Fresh and citrusy top notes, a hint of green, with a warm floral undertone

GEOGRAPHICAL ORIGIN
Italy, Morocco

SAFETY NOTES
Nontoxic, nonirritant

PROPERTIES
Skin rejuvenating, scar healing, antispasmodic, antidepressant

KEY USE
Skin care: for dry, sensitive, mature skin, scar tissue

OTHER USES
Stomach cramps, indigestion, irritable bowel syndrome, colitis

PSYCHOLOGICALLY
Excellent mental destressor, good for panic and shock

BLENDS WITH
Frankincense, Rose, Lavender, Lemon, Patchouli, Sandalwood

Soothing
Wedding-day nerves were once alleviated by using Neroli in the bride's bouquet.

Orange leaves
Petitgrain is an essential oil from the leaves of the bitter orange tree.

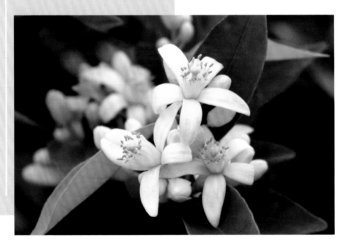

Essential Oils for the Muscles & Circulation

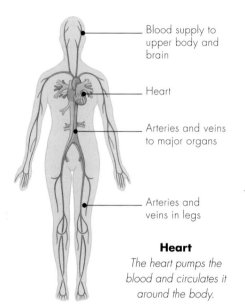

Blood supply to upper body and brain

Heart

Arteries and veins to major organs

Arteries and veins in legs

Heart
The heart pumps the blood and circulates it around the body.

Essential oils are effective in helping problems linked to the circulation and the musculoskeletal system. They are best applied using massage techniques or in a bath, both of which allow the oils to penetrate the skin.

Warming oils

Many essential oils are warming, easing out stiffness in the muscles and improving poor circulation, which shows on the skin as a reddening effect and a tingling sensation. Cold hands and feet, another sign of poor circulation, are helped by massaging in blends of warming oils, such as Rosemary or Ginger. These oils also help to remove toxins from the areas that are massaged.

Anti-inflammatory oils

Some essential oils also have a mild anti-inflammatory effect, useful for pain relief and swelling and helpful for injuries or strained muscles.

High blood pressure

Gentle massage and blends of relaxing oils are useful for people who are suffering from high blood pressure or increased pulse due to stress, pressure, or anxiety. But remember, if you are using essential oils on someone with high blood pressure, be careful to use low concentrations of soothing oils, and avoid stimulating blends and deep massages.

Cellulite

Cellulite is an accumulation of water and toxic waste in the fatty layer under the skin, which causes hard lumps to form, and gives the skin an "orange peel" look. This is best treated by a qualified therapist who knows how to deliver a deep, detoxifying massage to the area. There is no quick fix, and along with aromatherapy treatment you also need to undertake a detoxifiying routine by adopting a wholefood diet, removing caffeine, giving up smoking, getting regular exercise, and massaging yourself daily with a blend of detoxifying oils, for at least two months. It takes discipline.

To make a good anticellulite blend, mix 3 drops Juniper, 4 drops Lemon, and 3 drops Fennel in 4 teaspoons (20 milliliters) of sweet almond oil. Massage the blend into the affected area twice daily.

Key Essential Oil

Rosemary is very warming and stimulating to aching muscles.

49

CYPRESS *Cupressus sempervirens*

The strengthening and fortifying fragrance of cypress has long been used as an incense in the Far East. In Ancient Greece, cypress trees were said to be the gateways to the Underworld. Nicholas Culpeper (1616–1654), one of the fathers of Western herbal medicine, used cypress to check excess fluids in the body. The sharp green fragrance is used in many perfume formulas.

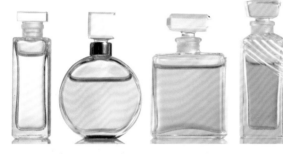

Perfume
Cypress is used in men's and women's fragrances.

Datafile

BOTANICAL NAME
Cupressus sempervirens

PLANT TYPE
Evergreen tree with small, brownish cones

OIL FROM
Needles and twigs

FRAGRANCE
Strong, sharp, and green, slightly smoky with a hint of sweetness

GEOGRAPHICAL ORIGIN
France, Spain

SAFETY NOTES
Nontoxic, nonirritant

PROPERTIES
Local circulation stimulant, detoxifying, antiseptic, antispasmodic

KEY USE
Muscular and circulatory: aches and pains, cramps, poor circulation, fluid retention

OTHER USES
Spasmodic coughs, bronchitis, oily skin, infected cuts

PSYCHOLOGICALLY
Calms the breathing and relieves anxiety

BLENDS WITH
Atlas Cedarwood, Lemon, Rosemary, Lemongrass, Juniper

ROSEMARY

Rosmarinus officinalis This is Shakespeare's herb of remembrance, mentioned by Ophelia in *Hamlet*. The bright, strong fragrance of rosemary is very stimulating to the mind. Sprigs of rosemary were burned as incense in Ancient Greece; the smoke is highly scented. A modern equivalent is to place sprigs of rosemary on the barbecue to flavor the cooking. A few drops on a tissue in the car helps concentration.

Datafile

BOTANICAL NAME
Rosmarinus officinalis

PLANT TYPE
Evergreen shrub with spiky leaves, and blue flowers

OIL FROM
Leaves and twigs

FRAGRANCE
Fresh, piney, with warm woody notes underneath

GEOGRAPHICAL ORIGIN
France, Spain, Tunisia

SAFETY NOTES
Generally nontoxic, nonirritant. Not advised for epileptics, people with high blood pressure, and pregnant women

PROPERTIES
Antispasmodic, analgesic, local circulation stimulant, antiseptic, expectorant

KEY USE
Muscular and circulatory: aches and pains, backache, poor circulation, rheumatism, fluid retention

OTHER USES
Scalp tonic to promote hair growth, coughs, colds, flu, lethargy

PSYCHOLOGICALLY
An invigorating fragrance that improves concentration and wakes up the brain

BLENDS WITH
Lemongrass, Vetiver, Ginger, Black Pepper, Lavender

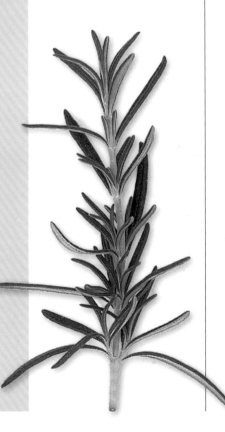

Oils for Muscles & Circulation • 1

Muscular Conditions & Treatments

The numbers next to the oils refer to the number of drops to be used. Halve the number of drops used on children between three and ten years of age.

CONDITION	OILS	METHOD
Aches and pains: after sports or gardening, for example	3 Ginger 4 Lavender	These essential oils in a hot bath at night will ease pain and help sleep
Muscular stiffness	3 Vetiver 3 Lavender 4 Ginger	These essential oils in 4 teaspoons (20 milliliters) of sweet almond oil. Apply half a teaspoonful twice a day to the affected areas
Cramps: strain due to overuse of muscles	4 Lavender 4 Rosemary	Apply an ice-cold compress twice daily until pain eases
Backache: pain, stiffness, and poor circulation	4 Ginger 2 Vetiver	These essential oils in 4 teaspoons (20 milliliters) of sweet almond oil. Massage in well twice daily to ease stiffness
Poor muscle tone: after a fracture, when the plaster cast has been removed, for example	4 Rosemary 4 Ginger 2 Lavender	These essential oils in 4 teaspoons (20 milliliters) of sweet almond oil. Massage one teaspoonful into the affected muscles twice daily to improve circulation and increase muscle mass
Sprain: torn or pulled ligaments, for example in the ankle	2 Peppermint 2 Lavender	Apply an ice-cold compress to the affected area, with the limb elevated, twice daily until swelling eases

Arthritis

There are different types of arthritic conditions that need specific types of care. If you are in any doubt about the appropriate treatment, consult your doctor.

Osteoarthritis is caused by the wear and tear of the joints, and is common in older age, bringing stiffness, pain, and poor circulation. A warming blend is needed, so use 4 drops Black Pepper, 4 drops Lavender, and 2 drops Vetiver in 4 teaspoons (20 milliliters) of sweet almond oil. Massage in half a teaspoonful to the affected area twice daily.

With rheumatoid arthritis, the joints are red and swollen, and they tend to flare up. There may also be general aches and pains and weakness. An anti-inflammatory blend of essential oils may be very gently applied— the use of a massage is not advised. Try 5 drops Roman Chamomile and 5 drops Lavender in 4 teaspoons (20 milliliters) of base lotion.

Key Essential Oil

Ginger essential oil has a warming effect on stiff joints and can be used to help muscular aches.

LEMONGRASS *Cymbopogon citratus* Lemongrass is a highly fragrant grass from India; in traditional medicine in India it is used to help treat fevers and infections. The oil is a very useful insect repellent, helpful for travelers or those living in hot climates. Try two drops of Lemongrass in a vaporizer to keep mosquitoes away. It is also used as a natural flavoring ingredient in nonalcoholic drinks.

Datafile

BOTANICAL NAME
Cymbopogon citratus

PLANT TYPE
Aromatic, tropical grass

OIL FROM
Fresh chopped grass

FRAGRANCE
Strong, lemony, zesty with heavy, slightly earthy undertone

GEOGRAPHICAL ORIGIN
India

SAFETY NOTES
Not advised for use on children or people with sensitive or damaged skin

PROPERTIES
Analgesic, local circulation stimulant, digestive tonic

KEY USE
Muscular and circulatory: aches and pains, cramps, strains, poor circulation and muscle tone

OTHER USES
Indigestion, colitis, sluggish digestion

PSYCHOLOGICALLY
Bright and uplifting, helpful as an antidepressant to lift your mood

BLENDS WITH
Frankincense, Rosemary, Ginger, Vetiver, Sandalwood, Peppermint

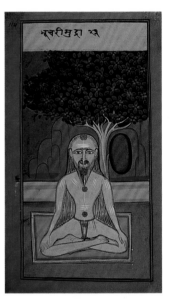

India
Powerful exotic fragrances come from India.

JUNIPER *Juniperus communis*

A jam made of Juniper berries is still eaten in Switzerland to help protect against chest infections and colds. Juniper oil is also the classic flavoring used in gin. This oil is a powerful diuretic. It takes two years for the juniper berries to mature ready for distillation. The berry oil is superior to oil from the wood or twigs.

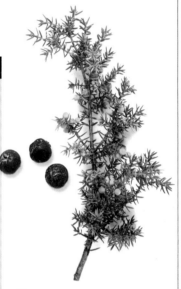

Datafile

BOTANICAL NAME
Juniperus communis

PLANT TYPE
Evergreen shrub which can grow up to 20 feet (6 meters) in height

OIL FROM
Ripe, black berries

FRAGRANCE
Pungent, green and piney-fresh with woody undertones

GEOGRAPHICAL ORIGIN
Central Europe

SAFETY NOTES
Generally nontoxic, not advised during pregnancy, or for those with kidney problems

PROPERTIES
Antispasmodic, local circulation stimulant, detoxifying, diuretic, antiseptic

KEY USE
Muscular and circulatory: aches and pains, cramps, cellulite, fluid retention, gout

OTHER USES
Weight loss, colds, the flu, oily complexion, lethargy

PSYCHOLOGICALLY
An uplifting and fortifying fragrance, good for mental fatigue and anxiety.

BLENDS WITH
Lemon, Fennel, Eucalyptus, Rosemary, Cypress

Cleanser
The Ancient Egyptians used Juniper to combat disease.

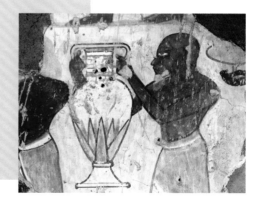

Oils for Muscles
& Circulation • 2

Muscular & Circulatory Conditions & Treatments

The numbers next to the oils refer to the number of drops to be used. Halve the number of drops used for children between three and ten years of age.

CONDITION	OILS	METHOD
Poor circulation: noticeable by cold extremities	3 Ginger 3 Black Pepper	These essential oils in a comfortably warm bath. Brush the skin first to boost circulation
Low blood pressure: lethargy, weakness, chilly limbs, dizziness on rising. If symptoms persist seek medical advice	3 Vetiver 2 Lemongrass 5 Rosemary	These essential oils in 4 teaspoons (20 milliliters) of grapeseed oil. Apply a full body massage at least once a week to boost the circulation and tone the body
Edema: fluid retention. If symptoms persist seek medical advice	3 Juniper 4 Lemon 3 Fennel	These diuretic essential oils in 4 teaspoons (20 milliliters) of sweet almond oil. Massage into the affected areas with upward strokes, toward the heart
Lymphatic congestion: toxin build-up, low energy	4 Fennel 2 Juniper 4 Cypress	These essential oils in 4 teaspoons (20 milliliters) of grapeseed oil. Massage one teaspoonful into lower legs and feet at least twice a week. Eat a diet rich in fresh foods and exercise in the fresh air
Gout: build-up of uric acid in the tissues, creating crystal deposits around joints	4 Juniper 6 Roman Chamomile	These essential oils in 4 teaspoons (20 milliliters) of base lotion. Apply very gently to the affected area. Avoid deep massages

Palpitations, High Blood Pressure & Varicose Veins

An increase in heart rate, especially stress-induced, more frequently than normal is cause for concern and should be medically investigated. A bath with 4 drops Lavender and 3 drops Neroli is calming.

Those with high blood pressure do benefit from a gentle massage; on no account should a deep massage be given. In 4 teaspoons (20 milliliters) of grapeseed oil, blend 7 drops Sandalwood and 3 drops Ylang Ylang. Apply one teaspoonful a day in a relaxing neck and shoulder massage.

Varicose veins can benefit from the gentle application of a cooling lotion; however, on no account massage an affected area. To 4 teaspoons (20 milliliters) of base lotion add 5 drops Roman Chamomile and 5 drops Palmarosa.

Key Essential Oil

Ylang Ylang is calming and destressing for states of anxiety.

FRENCH MARJORAM *Origanum marjorana* Sweet marjoram is a well-known herb, used in cooking and medicine. Warming and soothing, it is very helpful for worry and nervous tension. It is easy to grow in a sunny, well-drained soil. In the past, "swete bags" for the bath, filled with the herb, were used as personal hygiene products.

Datafile

BOTANICAL NAME
Origanum marjorana

PLANT TYPE
Bushy herb with green oval leaves and tiny, grayish-white flowers

OIL FROM
Dried herb

FRAGRANCE
Sharp, herbal, and medicinal, with a warm woody undertone

GEOGRAPHICAL ORIGIN
Mediterranean regions

SAFETY NOTES
Nontoxic, nonsensitizing

PROPERTIES
Antispasmodic, analgesic, antiseptic, hypotensive, menstrual tonic

KEY USE
Muscular: aches and pains, backache, stiffness, arthritis

OTHER USES
Headaches, migraines, menstrual cramps, constipation, stomach cramps

PSYCHOLOGICALLY
Warming and grounding, useful for insomnia and anxiety

BLENDS WITH
Lavender, Sandalwood, Patchouli, Orange, Roman Chamomile

VETIVER *Vetiveria zizanoides*

In India, mats are woven out of the grassy tops of vetiver. It is known in the East as the "oil of tranquility." Its deeply smoky, earthy fragrance is very emotionally stabilizing. It is used by the perfumery industry as a base note in fragrances for men and women. In aromatherapy it is a powerful destressor.

Datafile

BOTANICAL NAME
Vetiveria zizanoides

PLANT TYPE
Tall scented grass with strongly fragranced roots

OIL FROM
Roots

FRAGRANCE
Earthy, sensual, warm, and smoky

GEOGRAPHICAL ORIGIN
Java, Haiti, Reunion

SAFETY NOTES
Nontoxic, nonirritant

PROPERTIES
Antispasmodic, local circulation stimulant, nervous sedative

KEY USE
Muscular: aches and pains, backache, stiffness, arthritis

OTHER USES
Menstrual cramps, stomach cramps

PSYCHOLOGICALLY
Deeply comforting and strengthening, for states of depression and anxiety, and for sexual insecurities

BLENDS WITH
Neroli, Jasmine, Patchouli, Rose, Lavender, Petitgrain

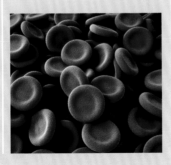

Red blood cells
Vetiver is warming to the circulation.

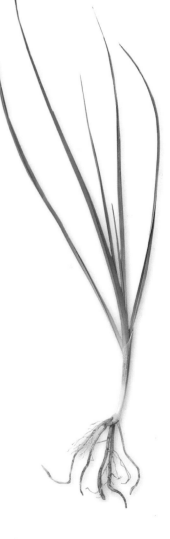

Essential Oils for the Respiratory System

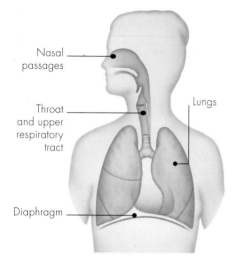

Nasal passages

Throat and upper respiratory tract

Lungs

Diaphragm

Inhalation
When inhaled, essential oils quickly reach the respiratory passages.

Essential oils can be used very effectively to treat problems in the respiratory tract. Many of the most useful oils, such as Eucalyptus, have a powerful vapor that, when inhaled, helps to ease mucous deposits out of the chest and loosen coughs to make them more productive. Other, gentler oils deepen the breathing and ease spasm in the respiratory passages.

Using the oils

Methods of using the oils need to be varied in order to achieve the best effects. Vaporizers, either electrical or flame driven, can be placed in the bedroom or the workspace to provide a background fragrance of useful decongestant oils. Baths are very useful nighttime treatments, and lying in the hot water and breathing in the gentle vapor will bring relaxation and ease, as well as ensuring that you get a good night's sleep.

Chest rubs are blends that are specifically applied to the chest, morning and night, to help breathing and ease congestion. Rub them in well and cover the area with a warm scarf. Finally, footbaths work very well to help shivers and chills. Soak the feet for 20 minutes and wrap up warmly.

The classic way to do an inhalation is to lean over a bowl of boiling water with your head under a towel, and breathe in deeply inhaling oils such as Eucalyptus and Lemon (3 drops of each). It is also possible to buy vaporizing cups with a mask attachment, which makes the whole process simpler and less messy, and also makes it possible for inhalations to be done in the workplace if necessary. Look out for these in your local pharmacy.

Inhalation Points to Note

Steam from boiling water can scald the respiratory tract so always let the water cool for a minute or two before you begin.

Inhalations are not advised for asthmatics because the vapor is too intense.

Remove glasses or contact lenses.

Lift the towel occasionally to aid breathing.

If you are treating children, supervise them constantly.

Key Essential Oil

Eucalyptus is a classic oil for chesty coughs and colds, the flu, and aching muscles.

EUCALYPTUS *Eucalyptus globulus*

Eucalyptus is a powerful antiseptic chest remedy from Australia, familiar as an ingredient in many pharmaceutical preparations for colds, the flu, or aching muscles. There are approximately 700 species of eucalyptus, of which this, the *globulus*, or Blue Gum, is the most commonly used in aromatherapy. The fragrance is instantly clearing.

Datafile

BOTANICAL NAME
Eucalyptus globulus

PLANT TYPE
Tall evergreen tree with blue-green leaves and a smooth, pale bark

OIL FROM
Leaves and young twigs

FRAGRANCE
Strong, medicinal, and sharp, with a woody undertone

GEOGRAPHICAL ORIGIN
Australia, China

SAFETY NOTES
Nontoxic, nonsensitizing. Do not use on infants and small children

PROPERTIES
Antiseptic, expectorant, decongestant, local circulation stimulant

KEY USE
Respiratory: colds, the flu, coughs, bronchitis

OTHER USES
Muscular aches and pains, osteoarthritis, skin infections

PSYCHOLOGICALLY
Clearing, fresh, and bright, gives a feeling of space

BLENDS WITH
Lemon, Peppermint, Tea Tree, Atlas Cedarwood

First aid
Eucalyptus should be a key ingredient in home first-aid kits.

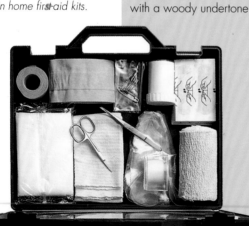

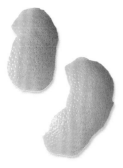

LEMON *Citrus limonum* Lemon is very popular in Mediterranean countries as a tonic for infectious illness. A wonderful zesty oil is produced in Sicily. The oil is pressed from the peel of the fruit, and if you scrape a thin piece from the rind of a lemon and turn it over, you can clearly see the little oil-filled sacs in the peel.

Datafile

BOTANICAL NAME
Citrus limonum

PLANT TYPE
Small evergreen tree with very fragrant flowers and succulent, ripe yellow fruit

OIL FROM
Fruit peel

FRAGRANCE
Bright, fresh, sherbety sweet

GEOGRAPHICAL ORIGIN
Mediterranean regions

SAFETY NOTES
Phototoxic. Do not expose skin to ultraviolet (UV) light for 12 hours after the application of a blend

PROPERTIES
Antiseptic, immune-boosting, detoxifying, expectorant, antidepressant

KEY USE
Respiratory: colds, the flu, sinusitis, bronchitis, chest infections

OTHER USES
Oily skin, acne, osteoarthritis, lymphatic congestion, lethargy

PSYCHOLOGICALLY
Antidepressant, uplifting, improves well-being

BLENDS WITH
Lavender, Peppermint, Atlas Cedarwood, Neroli, Patchouli

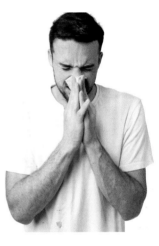

Cold remedy
Lemon is widely used in remedies for coughs, colds, and the flu.

Oils for Respiratory Problems • 1

Respiratory Conditions & Treatments

The numbers next to the oils refer to the number of drops to be used. Use half the number of stated drops for sensitive skin, or children between three and ten years old.

CONDITION	OILS	METHOD
Bronchitis: chest infection following cold or the flu	4 Tea Tree 4 Atlas Cedarwood	Inhalation, twice a day
	5 Tea Tree 5 Eucalyptus	These essential oils in 4 teaspoons (20 milliliters) of grapeseed oil, to make a chest rub. Apply half a teaspoonful to the affected area morning and night
Sinusitis: blocked and painful sinuses, a green or bright yellow discharge	4 Tea Tree 2 Peppermint	Inhalation, twice a day
	6 Tea Tree 4 Lemon	These essential oils in 4 teaspoons (20 milliliters) of grapeseed oil. Apply half a teaspoonful to the face with a very gentle massage, especially at night
Dry cough: sore, tickly, and nonproductive	2 Sandalwood 4 Atlas Cedarwood	Inhalation, morning and night
Mucous cough: clear white or greenish discharge	4 Tea Tree 4 Eucalyptus 2 Peppermint	These essential oils in 20 milliliters (4 teaspoons) of sweet almond oil to make a chest rub. Apply half a teaspoonful to the chest, morning and night
Throat infection: soreness, difficulty swallowing	2 Sandalwood	Apply neat to outside of throat, rub in gently. A gargle also helps. Sprinkle the essential oil into a tumbler of warm water and stir well. Take a mouthful, gargle, and spit out

Asthma

Constriction of the airways, making the chest tight and breathing difficult, is worrying, especially in the young. Aromatherapy can help, but it is important not to discontinue any medication prescribed by your doctor. Using a vaporizer with 2 drops Atlas Cedarwood and 4 drops Lavender at night will help sleep. The same oils can also be used in the bath. Remember to halve the quantities for children.

Lavender is one of the best oils to use for asthma; it is relaxing and calming emotionally, and a gentle antispasmodic that soothes and comforts distress. Frankincense and Atlas Cedarwood are woody, comforting oils that help slow down the breathing, giving a sense of peace and openness to the chest.

Treating Children

Children aged between three and ten can be treated for the conditions described on page 64, but half the number of stated drops must be used. A vaporizer in the bedroom with 3 drops Eucalyptus and 3 drops Lavender will aid sleep.

Key Essential Oil

Atlas Cedarwood helps to calm breathing, used in a vaporizer.

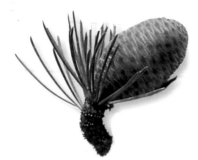

ATLAS CEDARWOOD *Cedrus atlantica*

This oil comes from a beautiful majestic tree that can grow up to 130 feet (40 meters) in height. It has a sweeping, tentlike appearance. Standing within its canopy, looking up at the enormous trunk, surrounded by the fragrance of the wood, brings a deeply meditative experience.

Datafile

BOTANICAL NAME
Cedrus atlantica

PLANT TYPE
Tall evergreen with reddish, aromatic wood

OIL FROM
Wood

FRAGRANCE
Medicinal top note with warm, sweet, woody undertone

GEOGRAPHICAL ORIGIN
Atlas Mountains in North Africa

SAFETY NOTES
Nontoxic, nonirritant. Not advised during pregnancy

PROPERTIES
Expectorant, antispasmodic, skin rejuvenating, nervous sedative

KEY USE
Respiratory: coughs, bronchitis, chest infections, asthma

OTHER USES
Weeping eczema, mature skin, dandruff, acne

PSYCHOLOGICALLY
Destressing, calming, soothing, good for anxiety

BLENDS WITH
Frankincense, Rose, Patchouli, Eucalyptus, Lemon

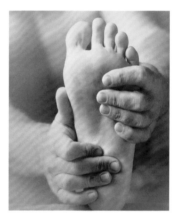

Feet
Atlas Cedarwood can help to heal cracked skin on the heels.

SANDALWOOD *Santalum album* With

thousands of years of use behind it, this beautiful oil comes originally from India. It takes around 30 years for the tree to mature to produce high quality oil. The oil is highly prized in India as a medicinal tonic, a sacred incense, and a perfume ingredient. The rich aroma appeals to both men and women.

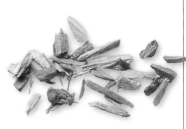

Datafile

BOTANICAL NAME
Santalum album

PLANT TYPE
Small evergreen tree with scented heartwood

OIL FROM
Wood

FRAGRANCE
Soft, sweet, and rich with warm, woody, spicy undertones

GEOGRAPHICAL ORIGIN
India

SAFETY NOTES
Nontoxic, nonirritant

PROPERTIES
Expectorant, antiseptic, skin rejuvenating, genitourinary tonic

KEY USE
Respiratory: dry and mucous coughs, sore throats, bronchitis

OTHER USES
Acne, oily skin, mature skin, cystitis, candida

PSYCHOLOGICALLY
Deeply relaxing and calming. Good for anxiety, depression, and insomnia

BLENDS WITH
Benzoin, Rose, Neroli, Lemon, Patchouli Atlas Cedarwood

Calm
The soft, woody fragrance of Sandalwood can assist meditation.

Oils for Respiratory Problems • 2

Respiratory Conditions & Treatments

The numbers next to the oils refer to the number of drops to be used. Use half the number of stated drops for sensitive skin, or children between three and ten years old.

CONDITION	OILS	METHOD
Tonsillitis: inflammation of the tonsils, at the back of the throat, with a headache, fever, or earache. Seek medical attention	3 Tea Tree 3 Eucalyptus	Aromatherapy can help support the immune system during the period of infection. Use these essential oils in a vaporizer in the bedroom
Whooping cough: seek medical attention	3 Eucalyptus 3 Atlas Cedarwood	Aromatherapy plays a supportive role here. Use these oils in a vaporizer to assist breathing. A warm bath with 2 drops Lavender will aid sleep
Hay fever: allergic reaction in the nose and airways in response to pollen, dust, fungus, or animal fur	2 Peppermint 4 Lavender	Vaporize these essential oils to ease the breathing or sniff on a tissue
Chronic phlegm: in some people this is always present, and is a sign of low immunity and poor elimination	2 Rosemary 2 Peppermint	Sprinkle these essential oils on a tissue and sniff to loosen congestion in the daytime
Laryngitis: inflammation of the vocal chords due to infection, leading to barking cough and possibly loss of voice	2 Tea Tree 2 Eucalyptus 2 Sandalwood	Inhale 2–3 times daily to soothe the throat

Colds & Flu

If either a cold or the flu threatens, first try taking an immune-boosting evening bath with 2 drops Tea Tree, 2 drops Black Pepper, and 2 drops Bergamot. Repeat this each night, and rest as much as possible. Vaporize 3 drops Tea Tree and 3 drops Eucalyptus to disinfect the air. Make up a chest rub by blending 4 drops Tea Tree, 2 drops Sandalwood, and 4 drops Lemon in 4 teaspoons (20 milliliters) of sweet almond oil. Apply half a teaspoonful to the throat and chest twice daily.

Aromatherapy helps to encourage rest and relaxation, bringing ease to congested noses throats, and chests, and if used consistently can keep the period of infection to a minimum.

Key Essential Oil

Lemon essential oil is a good booster of the immune system.

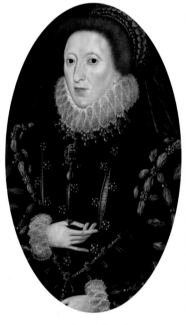

BENZOIN *Styrax benzoin*

In the Far East, benzoin is highly prized as an incense and medicine. In the West it is used in a remedy called Friar's balsam, an old-fashioned respiratory tonic. In the 16th century, Queen Elizabeth the first of England was fond of its fragrance. Then it was known as gum benjamin. In aromatherapy it is also valued as a destressor.

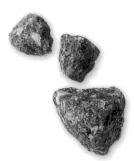

Royal application

Benzoin was a favorite scent of Queen Elizabeth I.

Datafile

BOTANICAL NAME
Styrax benzoin

PLANT TYPE
Tropical tree, which produces the gum in response to damage or cuts in its bark made deliberately to encourage secretion

OIL FROM
Gum, however, benzoin is a resinoid, not an essential oil, that is dissolved out of the gum using solvents

FRAGRANCE
Sweet, rich, and vanilla-like

GEOGRAPHICAL ORIGIN
Sumatra

SAFETY NOTES
Not advised for people with allergy-prone skin

PROPERTIES
Expectorant, antiseptic, healing, nervous sedative

KEY USE
Respiratory: coughs, colds, bronchitis, chest infections

OTHER USES
Cuts, grazes, cracked heels, chapped skin

PSYCHOLOGICALLY
Very calming, soothing, antidepressant, nurturing

BLENDS WITH
Lemon, Atlas Cedarwood, Frankincense, Lavender, Sandalwood

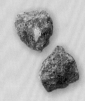

TEA TREE *Melaleuca alternifolia* Tea Tree oil is one of the biggest successes in aromatherapy, now widely used in a whole range of cosmetic and dental products. It is native to Australia, mainly to New South Wales, and was traditionally used as a remedy by the Aboriginal people. As an antiseptic, antifungal, and antiviral oil it covers a very broad spectrum of use—don't leave home without it.

Versatility
Tea Tree has a wide range of applications.

Datafile

BOTANICAL NAME
Melaleuca alternifolia

PLANT TYPE
Small tree with fine, needle-like leaves

OIL FROM
Leaves and twigs

FRAGRANCE
Strongly medicinal, clear, green, and fresh

GEOGRAPHICAL ORIGIN
Australia

SAFETY NOTES
Nontoxic, nonirritant

PROPERTIES
Antiseptic, antibacterial, antifungal, expectorant, antiviral

KEY USE
Respiratory: colds, the flu, bronchitis, whooping cough

OTHER USES
Athlete's foot, candida, nailbed infections, infected cuts, wounds. This oil can be used neat on the skin

PSYCHOLOGICALLY
Fresh and vitalizing, strengthens the spirit

BLENDS WITH
Bergamot, Black Pepper, Ginger, Lavender, Atlas Cedarwood

Respiratory

Nailbed Infections

Candida

Cuts

Athlete's Foot

Essential Oils for Digestion

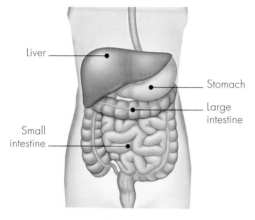

Digestion

Efficient digestion is vital to health.

Aromatherapy can be of great assistance in treating digestive problems. We take in foods of varying types and quality every day, yet are completely unaware of our digestive tract, busy extracting the nutrients and converting them for our use.

Tone up

We are often erratic in our eating patterns, and experience problems such as constipation because our digestion is sluggish. Essential oils can really help tone up the digestion, to improve the rhythm of elimination, and to ease the underlying stress that can so often be an issue. Stress can quickly affect the digestive process, and abdominal massage, either self-applied or by a professional, can quickly relieve muscular tension in the abdomen.

Eating habits

Poor eating habits can have a negative psychological impact on the system too. Eating meals when stressed, under pressure, angry, or while watching destructive images on television does not help to create relaxed digestion. Also, a sedentary lifestyle with little exercise does not stimulate enough rhythm in the large intestine to encourage regular elimination.

Try to achieve a balance between rest, relaxation, a healthy wholefood diet, regular exercise, and a positive attitude. Essential oils such as Black Pepper, Ginger, Peppermint, Lemongrass, Orange, or Roman Chamomile can all be used to help warm and soothe the abdominal area, and also have the effect of stimulating the appetite.

Safety

It is important to stress that essential oils are not swallowed or taken orally. The lining of the digestive tract is extremely sensitive, and would be damaged by oral dosage. Essential oils can be used very effectively in a massage or in the bath to treat digestive problems.

There have been a number of cases of poisoning with large doses of essential oils that have been swallowed, sometimes by accident, so keep all essential oils out of the reach of children.

For children aged between three and ten, please halve any stated number of drops in a blend in the same amount of carrier product.

Key Essential Oil

Peppermint essential oil refreshes and eases the process of digestion.

PEPPERMINT
Mentha piperita In Ancient Greece, wreaths of peppermint were worn on the head at feasts, and tables were decorated with it. In England, in the 18th century, there were famous peppermint fields in Mitcham, in Surrey. Nowadays, most of the oil comes from the United States and is used to flavor toothpaste and chewing gum.

Datafile

BOTANICAL NAME
Mentha piperita

PLANT TYPE
Vigorous herb with fresh, minty scented leaves

OIL FROM
Leaves

FRAGRANCE
Powerfully fresh, sharp, and cooling

GEOGRAPHICAL ORIGIN
United States

SAFETY NOTES
Nontoxic, however, this is a strong oil so use in low concentration. Not advised for people with high blood pressure, pregnant women, infants, and small children

PROPERTIES
Analgesic, antispasmodic, expectorant, decongestant

KEY USE
Digestive: indigestion, irritable bowel syndrome, constipation

OTHER USES
Muscular aches, cramps, osteoarthritis, coughs, sinusitis

PSYCHOLOGICALLY
Invigorating and bright, helps headaches and mental stress

BLENDS WITH
Lemon, Ginger, Black Pepper, Fennel, Lemongrass, Rosemary

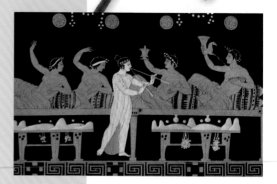

Greece
The Ancient Greeks loved Peppermint at their feasts.

BLACK PEPPER *Piper nigrum* In ancient times, black pepper was considered so valuable that 3,000 pounds of it was demanded in ransom for the city of Rome. Familiar as a flavoring on the dining table, its use as an essential oil may come as quite a surprise, but it is one of the best warming oils for the digestion and circulation.

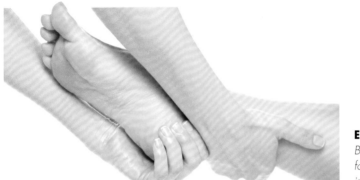

Extremities
Black Pepper is useful for improving the circulation in the hands and feet.

Datafile

BOTANICAL NAME
Piper nigrum

PLANT TYPE
Climbing vine with beautiful, heart-shaped green leaves and clusters of flowers that ripen into the fruit

OIL FROM
Crushed and dried black peppercorns

FRAGRANCE
Musty, spicy, sharp with underlying sweetness

GEOGRAPHICAL ORIGIN
India

SAFETY NOTES
Nontoxic, nonirritant

PROPERTIES
Analgesic, local circulation stimulant, antispasmodic, expels wind, immune tonic

KEY USE
Digestive: stomach cramps, indigestion, irritable bowel syndrome, bloating, poor appetite, constipation

OTHER USES
Muscular aches, osteoarthritis, poor circulation, the flu, chills

PSYCHOLOGICALLY
Warming and aphrodisiac, good for impotence and sexual disharmony

BLENDS WITH
Fennel, Peppermint, Lemon, Bergamot, Tea Tree, Ginger, Lemongrass

Oils for Digestion • 1

Digestive Conditions & Treatments

The numbers next to the oils refer to the number of drops to be used. Halve the number of drops used for children between three and ten years of age.

CONDITION	OILS	METHOD
Indigestion: with abdominal pain, bloating, nausea	2 Peppermint 4 Black Pepper 4 Ginger	These essential oils in 4 teaspoons (20 milliliters) of grapeseed oil. Massage half a teaspoonful into the affected area three times daily
Constipation: irregular and difficult elimination of stools	2 Neroli 2 Peppermint 6 Black Pepper	These essential oils in 4 teaspoons (20 milliliters) of sweet almond oil. Massage half a teaspoonful into the abdomen with a circular motion from right to left, three times daily
Nausea: a feeling of sickness with dizziness and sweating	2 Peppermint or 2 Ginger	Sprinkle the oil on a tissue and sniff Sprinkle the oil on a tissue and sniff
Colic: this may involve waves of abdominal pain, possibly due to wind, constipation, or blockage of the bowel	4 Ginger 4 Lavender 2 Peppermint	These essential oils in 4 teaspoons (20 milliliters) of grapeseed oil. Massage gently over the abdomen, in a circular motion, and cover with a hot water bottle
Loss of appetite: perhaps due to illness or emotional stress	2 Neroli 2 Roman Chamomile 6 Bergamot 2 Neroli 2 Fennel	These essential oils in a warm bath is a gentle treatment These essential oils in 4 teaspoons (20 milliliters) of grapeseed oil. Massage gently into the abdomen

Irritable Bowel Syndrome

This is a condition very much on the increase. It is influenced by stress, and symptoms include alternating constipation and diarrhea, pain in the abdomen, and bloating. It is recommended that the diet of a sufferer be assessed by a nutritional expert, because dietary allergies may be causing the problems. Aromatherapy treatment from a professional is also advisable, especially in order to treat the underlying stress. A home blend of 2 drops Peppermint, 4 drops Ginger, and 4 drops Black Pepper in 4 teaspoons (20 milliliters) of grapeseed oil can be massaged over the abdomen three times daily, using a hot water bottle to bring warmth to the area and improve the absorption of the oils.

Safety for Children

For babies use one drop only of either Roman Chamomile or Lavender in 4 teaspoons (20 milliliters) of sweet almond oil for a very gentle abdominal massage.

Warning

Consult your doctor if you experience any undiagnosed change in bowel habits that persists for more than two weeks.

GINGER *Zingiber officinale*

Ginger has many thousands of years of use behind it as a medicine, tonic, and spice. It is a key ingredient in Chinese medicine for digestive complaints. The roots must be at least one year old before they contain the maximum amount of essential oil. Ginger tea, made from one teaspoonful of chopped root in boiling water, infused for ten minutes, is great for colds and the flu.

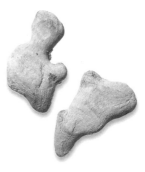

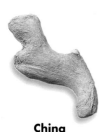

China

Ginger root has long been a favorite of the Chinese for its warm, pungent, and penetrating properties.

Datafile

BOTANICAL NAME
Zingiber officinale

PLANT TYPE
Tall plant with pairs of long dark green leaves and a thick, fleshy root

OIL FROM
Dried roots

FRAGRANCE
Warm, sweet, spicy, soft

GEOGRAPHICAL ORIGIN
China, India

SAFETY NOTES
Nontoxic, nonirritant

PROPERTIES
Analgesic, antispasmodic, expels gas, expectorant, immune tonic

KEY USE
Digestive: indigestion, colic, bloating, irritable bowel syndrome, constipation

OTHER USES
Muscular aches, lethargy, poor circulation, influenza, chesty coughs

PSYCHOLOGICALLY
Warming and energizing, good for lack of confidence and depression

BLENDS WITH
Lemon, Black Pepper, Lemongrass, Fennel, Orange

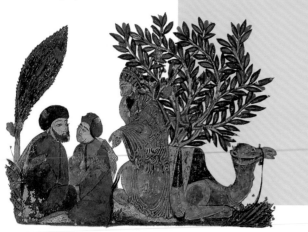

FENNEL *Foeniculum vulgare* In ancient times,

fennel was regarded as a tonic for eyestrain. It is also an ingredient in the original gripe water given to infants for flatulence and colic. Nicholas Culpeper, one of the fathers of Western herbal medicine, talks about fennel easing "painful windy swelling." In a blend massaged across the shoulders the essential oil can help promote breast milk flow.

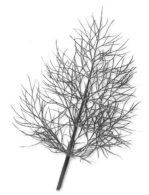

Baby oil
Fennel promotes breast milk and eases infant colic.

Datafile

BOTANICAL NAME
Foeniculum vulgare

PLANT TYPE
Herb. Grows up to 6 ½ feet (2 meters) in height, with wispy leaves and yellow flowers

OIL FROM
Seeds

FRAGRANCE
Sweet, aniseed, spicy

GEOGRAPHICAL ORIGIN
Central Europe

SAFETY NOTES
Nontoxic, nonirritant. Not advised for epileptics, people with kidney problems, pregnant women, infants, and small children

PROPERTIES
Antispasmodic, expels gas, expectorant, menstrual regulator, improves flow of breast milk

KEY USE
Digestive: stomach cramps, indigestion, irritable bowel syndrome, constipation

OTHER USES
Chesty coughs, period pains, menopause

PSYCHOLOGICALLY
Mentally refreshing, assists concentration

BLENDS WITH
Lemongrass, Ginger, Sandalwood, Geranium

Essential Oils for Genitourinary Health

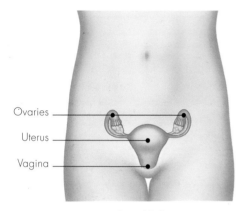

Sensitivity
Oils should be used with care in the genitourinary area.

Women's health

Aromatherapists find themselves very often dealing with women's health issues. The nature of aromatherapy treatment, combining nurturing touch and wonderful fragrances, makes a very positive contribution to energy levels, mental attitude, and overall well-being. There are very useful essential oils that will help to balance and regulate the menstrual cycle and deal with the symptoms of premenstrual syndrome. The effect is achieved as much through the psychological effects of the fragrances as it is through application.

For self-treatment, the ways to apply the oils are in baths and massages. The abdomen requires special attention, especially if there are menstrual cramps; gentle massage with a circular motion from right to left is soothing, and can be followed by a hot water bottle wrapped in a towel to bring warmth to the area.

Pregnancy & childbirth

As well as general gynecological issues, aromatherapy can help a great deal during pregnancy and after the birth, if the correct oils and techniques are used. It's important to use it with the support of your doctor, and preferably to receive treatment and advice from a qualified aromatherapist. You will find a section on applications and safety issues on pages 88–89, if you want to use oils on yourself.

Men's health

For men, the health of the genitourinary area is vital, and Indian and Chinese medicinal approaches are very aware of this fact. Issues in older men may well revolve around the health of the prostate gland, where infection and enlargement is very common, and an aromatherapy tonic can be very useful.

Treatment may also concentrate on issues around fertility, or sexual disharmony due to stress. Many men respond very well to Jasmine as a tonic to the sexual energies, with its deep and subtle fragrance helping to reassure the emotions, and Sandalwood to ground and stabilize feelings. Earthing and strengthening oils such as Patchouli and Vetiver ease anxiety, while Ginger can bring warmth and energy.

Key Essential Oil

Sandalwood essential oil is a gentle but effective genitourinary tonic.

PALMAROSA *Cymbopogon martini*

This tropical grass is a member of the same botanical family as lemongrass and citronella. It was originally native to India, although now much of the oil comes from Madagascar. The oil is wonderfully antiseptic and antifungal, with a sweet rosy aroma. It is very useful to have such a pleasant-smelling ingredient perform such a beneficial function.

Datafile

BOTANICAL NAME
Cymbopogon martini

PLANT TYPE
Tall grass with long slender stalks

OIL FROM
Dried grass

FRAGRANCE
Sweet, rosy, soft, slightly lemony

GEOGRAPHICAL ORIGIN
Madagascar

SAFETY NOTES
Nontoxic, nonirritant

PROPERTIES
Antiseptic, antifungal, skin regenerating, skin cooling, nervous sedative

KEY USE
Genitourinary: cystitis, vaginitis, yeast infections, premenstrual syndrome, menopausal hot flashes, mood swings, prostatitis

OTHER USES
Dry, sensitive, or mature skin, eczema, psoriasis, skin inflammation

PSYCHOLOGICALLY
Excellent for depression, anxiety, insomnia, and nervous exhaustion

BLENDS WITH
Fennel, Orange, Lemon, Lavender, Patchouli, Sandalwood

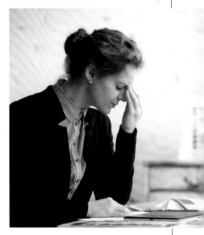

GERANIUM *Pelargonium graveolens* The finest geranium oil comes from the tropical island of Reunion, in the Pacific. Nicholas Culpeper, in his 17th-century herbal, refers to a wild species of geranium as being able to "expel the stone and gravel in the kidneys." The oil used in aromatherapy is noted for a cleansing and diuretic effect, as well as a regulating action on the skin, improving its suppleness.

Datafile

BOTANICAL NAME
Pelargonium graveolens

PLANT TYPE
Perennial shrub up to 3 feet (1 meter) in height with velvety, highly scented leaves

OIL FROM
Leaves

FRAGRANCE
Very sweet, roselike, slightly minty and lemony

GEOGRAPHICAL ORIGIN
Reunion (Pacific)

SAFETY NOTES
Nontoxic, nonirritant

PROPERTIES
Antiseptic, astringent, menstrual regulator, diuretic

KEY USE
Genitourinary: irregular periods, premenstrual syndrome, fluid retention, menopause

OTHER USES
Combination, dry, oily, and mature skin, acne, eczema

PSYCHOLOGICALLY
Antidepressant, uplifting, and mood enhancing. Particularly useful as a pre-menstrual oil to ease depression and emotional tension

BLENDS WITH
Sandalwood, Lemon, Lavender, Vetiver, Frankincense, Neroli

Uplifting
Geranium is commonly used to alleviate symptoms of depression.

Oils for Genitourinary Problems • 1

Genitourinary Conditions & Treatments

The numbers next to the oils refer to the number of drops to be used.

CONDITION	OILS	METHOD
Irregular periods: cycle has an erratic pattern	3 Fennel 4 Geranium 3 Vetiver	These essential oils in 4 teaspoons (20 milliliters) of sweet almond oil. Massage half a teaspoonful into the abdomen every night for three to four weeks
Period pain: cramps and spreading pain	5 Sweet Marjoram 3 Ginger 2 Vetiver	These essential oils in 4 teaspoons (20 milliliters) of grapeseed oil. Massage one teaspoonful into the abdomen three times daily, follow with a hot water bottle over the area
Premenstrual syndrome: to treat mood swings and depression	3 Lavender 3 Palmarosa	These essential oils in an evening bath
To treat breast tenderness and fluid retention	4 Geranium 4 Lavender 2 Roman Chamomile	These essential oils in 4 teaspoons (20 milliliters) of sweet almond oil. Massage a teaspoonful into the breasts and abdomen twice daily
Menstrual migraine	3 Sweet Marjoram 3 Lavender	Apply a cold compress to the head for 20 minutes
Cystitis: infection in the urinary tract, with pain on trying to urinate. If symptoms persist consult a doctor	3 Tea Tree 3 Sandalwood	These essential oils in a bath. Bathe twice a day

Menopause

This stage in a woman's life need not be a problem, in fact some women experience very few symptoms. Common issues, however, are mood swings, changes in energy levels, anxiety, loss of libido, and hot flashes. Aromatherapy concentrates on improving mood and energy, as well as providing hormone-balancing essential oils to the system. Rose is seen as one of the best oils to use at this time; it uplifts the emotions and symbolizes the feminine. In conjunction with Frankincense and Sandalwood, both tonic and uplifting, a beautiful blend can be made and applied at least once a week in a full body massage. Try 3 drops Rose, 3 drops Frankincense, and 4 drops Sandalwood in 4 teaspoons (20 milliliters) of sweet almond oil.

Vaginal Yeast Infections

This fungal infection requires bath treatment with 3 drops of Tea Tree and 3 drops Palmarosa in the evenings.

Key Essential Oil

Rose is a deeply feminine oil, a useful psychological support.

JASMINE *Jasminum officinale*

In traditional Western herbal medicine, jasmine was said to facilitate childbirth. It is prized in India as a perfume and a hair oil, and the flowers may also be woven into garlands and worn around the neck at religious ceremonies. The flowers are too delicate for distillation, so the solvent extraction process is used to provide jasmine absolute, which has a complex floral aroma.

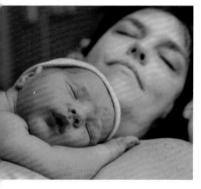

Delivery
Jasmine can help in childbirth.

Datafile

BOTANICAL NAME
Jasminum officinale

PLANT TYPE
Climbing shrub with elegant, delicate foliage and tiny, highly scented white flowers

OIL FROM
Flowers

FRAGRANCE
Extremely sweet, rich, heady, floral, and musky .

GEOGRAPHICAL ORIGIN
Morocco, Turkey

SAFETY NOTES
Nontoxic. Not be used during the first 8 months of pregnancy; it can be used to help childbirth

PROPERTIES
Antispasmodic, skin rejuvenating, helps labor, stimulates breast milk

KEY USE
Genitourinary: labor pains, lack of milk flow, menstrual cramps, impotence

OTHER USES
Asthma, coughs, dry or mature skin, dry hair and scalp

PSYCHOLOGICALLY
Deeply relaxing, sensual, for sexual disharmony and anxiety, also an aphrodisiac

BLENDS WITH
Clary Sage, Patchouli, Sandalwood, Frankincense, Orange

CLARY SAGE *Salvia sclarea* Nicholas Culpeper wrote, in his herbal of
1652, that clary sage "bringeth down women's courses and expelleth afterbirth,"
showing clearly its traditional use as an herb to encourage menstruation and help
childbirth symptoms. It is a handsome plant in an herb garden, with a pronounced
sweet, almost musky fragrance as you approach. The oil is noted for a very
pronounced mood-enhancing action, which brings a sense of euphoria.

Datafile

BOTANICAL NAME
Salvia sclarea

PLANT TYPE
Tall herb, up to 5 feet
(1.5 meters) in height, with
blueish-pink flowers

OIL FROM
Flowering tops and leaves

FRAGRANCE
Warm, nutty-sweet, green,
and soft

GEOGRAPHICAL ORIGIN
France

SAFETY NOTES
Nontoxic. Not advised during
pregnancy

PROPERTIES
Antispasmodic, menstrual
regulator, helps labor, skin
rejuvenating, lowers blood
pressure

KEY USE
Genitourinary: menstrual
cramps, irregular periods,
labor pains, menstrual
migraines, premenstrual
syndrome with mood swings

OTHER USES
Asthma, chesty
coughs, acne, dry skin,
dandruff, high blood
pressure

PSYCHOLOGICALLY
Calming and sedative, yet very
uplifting; cheers the mood

BLENDS WITH
Jasmine, Bergamot, Lavender,
Orange, Sandalwood

Oils for Pregnancy & Labor

The numbers next to the oils refer to the number of drops to be used.

CONDITION	OILS	METHOD
Morning sickness	1 Ginger	Sprinkle the essential oil on a tissue and sniff at intervals
Destress blend, three to nine months	2 Palmarosa 2 Neroli	These essential oils in 4 teaspoons (20 milliliters) of sweet almond oil. Let your partner massage your back, neck, and shoulders; sit on a stool and lean on a pillow on a table once you cannot lie on your front. Massage twice a week
Constipation	2 Ginger 2 Neroli	These essential oils in 4 teaspoons (20 milliliters) of sweet almond oil. Massage half a teaspoonful into the lower back with a circular motion, especially at night
Labor massage	2 Clary Sage 2 Jasmine	These essential oils in 4 teaspoons (20 milliliters) of grapeseed oil. In the early stages of labor, this blend can be massaged across the abdomen and lower back
Episiotomy stitches	3 Lavender	A warm bath will ease stinging and help healing

Safety While Pregnant

It is not advised to use essential oils on yourself in a massage for the first three months of your pregnancy. Carrier products such as jojoba or sweet almond oil can help stop stretch marks, but should be used unfragranced. After month three, you can add 4 drops Mandarin oil to 4 teaspoons (20 milliliters) of sweet almond oil, and massage half a teaspoonful in daily.

It is recommended that you avoid Jasmine and Clary Sage for the whole term of the pregnancy until labor, when they can be used.

Do not, at any time, consume essential oils by ingesting them through the mouth.

After the Birth

Gently massaging the lower back and abdomen after the birth helps settle the internal organs. Try 2 drops Rose and 2 drops Vetiver in 4 teaspoons (20 milliliters) sweet almond oil.

If breast milk is lacking, massage 2 drops Fennel and 2 drops Rose in 4 teaspoons (20 milliliters) of grapeseed oil over the shoulders and upper back, but not over the breast area.

For postpartum depression, try a weekly full body massage with 2 drops Neroli and 2 drops Rose in 4 teaspoons (20 milliliters) of sweet almond oil.

ROSE *Rosa damascena* "By any other name would smell as sweet" wrote Shakespeare; the sweet, heady fragrance of rose is famous as the symbol of true love. Candied rose petals, rose jam, and rosewater have been eaten and drunk since Roman times—what bliss to eat this divine aroma as well as be perfumed with it. It is the queen of essential oils, a deeply feminine aroma.

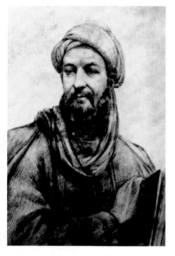

Ancient wisdom
The Islamic philosopher Avicenna distilled Rose in the 11th century.

Datafile

BOTANICAL NAME
Rosa damascena

PLANT TYPE
Shrub, up to 5 feet (1.5 meters) in height, with tiny, simple pink flowers

OIL FROM
Handpicked petals. An absolute is also produced by the solvent method

FRAGRANCE
The oil is soft, honey-sweet, very floral and slightly citrusy. The absolute is richer, more musky and spicy

GEOGRAPHICAL ORIGIN
The best oil is from the Kazanlik area in Bulgaria. The absolute often comes from Morocco

SAFETY NOTES
Nontoxic, nonirritant

PROPERTIES
Antispasmodic, menstrual regulator, liver tonic, skin rejuvenator

KEY USE
Genitourinary: irregular periods, premenstrual syndrome with mood swings, menopause, postpartum depression

OTHER USES
Sluggish digestion, dry, oily, or mature skin, eczema, cold sores

PSYCHOLOGICALLY
Good for deep-rooted feelings such as grief, anger, or helplessness. Wonderful for insomnia, anxiety, and mental tension

BLENDS WITH
Frankincense, Jasmine, Lemongrass, Vetiver, Patchouli, Mandarin

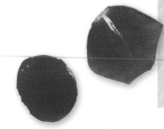

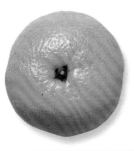

MANDARIN *Citrus reticulata*

This small citrus fruit has a traditional association with Christmas. The peel thrown on the fire creates a lovely, cheering fragrance. The oil is squeezed from the peel of the fruit, and is very safe to use with children, who love its sweetness. It has a bright aroma that is refreshing and encourages a positive mood in adults and children alike.

Datafile

BOTANICAL NAME
Citrus reticulata

PLANT TYPE
Evergreen tree up to 20 feet (6 meters) in height, with dark green leaves and fragrant flowers that ripen into fruit

OIL FROM
Peel of the fruit

FRAGRANCE
Sweet, citrus, fresh, and light

GEOGRAPHICAL ORIGIN
Southern Europe

SAFETY NOTES
Nontoxic, nonsensitizing. Phototoxic; do not expose skin to UV light for 12 hours after the application of a blend

PROPERTIES
Antispasmodic, nervous sedative, skin rejuvenating

KEY USE
Genitourinary: premenstrual syndrome with fluid retention, stretch marks in pregnancy

OTHER USES
Children's stomach upsets, constipation, dry, oily, or combination skin

PSYCHOLOGICALLY
Destressing, useful for children's upsets, anxieties, or sleeping problems. Also helps release inhibitions in adults

BLENDS WITH
Lavender, Lemon, Palmarosa, Neroli, Roman Chamomile

Skin
Mandarin oil is helpful for oily skin.

Essential Oils for the Nerves

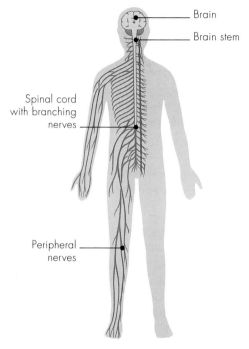

Nervous system
*From the spine nerve fibers
spread all over the body.*

Brain

Brain stem

Spinal cord
with branching
nerves

Peripheral
nerves

When there is too much to
do and too little time, when
it feels as though you are
pushing a boulder up a hill, when your
reserves are low and the slightest thing
sets you on edge, then you really need
aromatherapy.

Slow down

We become aware of nervous tension
through feelings of being on a short fuse,
through insomnia, or through shooting
pains like migraines. It is vital, at such
times, to stop. One of the best ways is
to take aromatherapy baths, especially
at night, using combinations of wonderful
destressing oils such as 4 drops of
Lavender and 2 drops Vetiver, or 4 drops
Bergamot and 2 drops Ylang Ylang. If
your routine is hectic, try to give yourself
30 minutes in the evening to unwind in
the bath. Use a vaporizer in the bedroom,
especially if you suffer from insomnia.
Leave it burning for 15 minutes before
you go to bed so the fragrance is in the
room when you settle down to sleep.

Migraines and headaches can be
helped by applying 4 drops of neat
Lavender to the forehead, temples, and
the back of the neck. A relaxing bath with
3 drops Sandalwood and 3 drops Neroli
will also calm anxiety or worry that may
underlie the headaches.

By consciously choosing to use
your favorite essential oils and simple
aromatherapy techniques such as baths,

or vaporizers, you will find that your lifestyle begins to shift to allow you more time and space to spend on yourself.

Jet Lag

Aromatherapy is increasingly being used to help with jet-lag symptoms. Essential oils can be used to help you stay awake, or relax you into sleep at times that are local to where you are, so that your body clock can adjust to the change in environment. Use a relaxing blend of 4 drops Sandalwood, 4 drops Lavender, and 2 drops Neroli in 4 teaspoons (20 milliliters) of carrier oil, applied after a bath or shower, to help you sleep. Or smell fresh zesty oils like Rosemary or Lemongrass; 2 drops of either oil on a tissue will help you stay awake until you can adjust to local time.

Key Essential Oil

Lavender dropped onto a tissue and sniffed helps nervousness before flying.

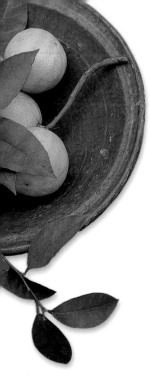

BERGAMOT *Citrus bergamia*
If you like the taste of Earl Grey tea, then you are aware of the fresh, citrusy perfume of this small bitter orange. The oil is an important ingredient in the original eau de cologne formula, which also includes Rosemary, Petitgrain, and Neroli, and is an old-fashioned remedy for stress and tension.

Datafile

BOTANICAL NAME
Citrus bergamia

PLANT TYPE
A variety of citrus tree grafted into bitter orange trees

OIL FROM
Peel of the fruit

FRAGRANCE
Fresh, soft, citrusy, and floral

GEOGRAPHICAL ORIGIN
Italy

SAFETY NOTES
Phototoxic. Do not expose the skin to ultraviolet (UV) rays for 12 hours after massaging a blend into the skin

PROPERTIES
Antidepressant, antiseptic, wound healing, digestive tonic, immune stimulant

KEY USE
Nervous system: anxiety, depression, mood swings, worry, insomnia

OTHER USES
Wounds, scar tissue, acne, indigestion, bloating, the flu, colds

PSYCHOLOGICALLY
Very uplifting, cheering, helps clear the clouds, soothes frustration

BLENDS WITH
Ylang Ylang, Frankincense, Lavender, Patchouli, Peppermint

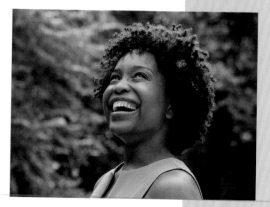

Mood-enhancing
Bergamot can lift the spirits for those suffering from depression.

YLANG YLANG *Cananga odorata* In Victorian times,
this oil was used in macassar oil, a treatment oil for the hair to give it shine. It is used by indigenous peoples in the tropics for the same purpose. The blooms are also used at their weddings, scattered on the marriage bed, no doubt because of its reputed aphrodisiac properties. Its aroma is heady and sweet.

Datafile

BOTANICAL NAME
Cananga odorata

PLANT TYPE
Tall tree with large, exotic yellow flowers high up in the canopy

OIL FROM
Flowers

FRAGRANCE
Very sweet, musky, soft, floral

GEOGRAPHICAL ORIGIN
Madagascar

SAFETY NOTES
Nontoxic, however, some people find the sweet fragrance causes a headache

PROPERTIES
Antidepressant, lowers blood pressure, nervous sedative, skin rejuvenator

KEY USE
Nervous system: anxiety, insomnia, depression, mood swings

OTHER USES
High blood pressure, rapid pulse, panic attacks, acne, oily skin

PSYCHOLOGICALLY
Deeply relaxing, destressing, soothes troubled mind and spirit. Thought to be an aphrodisiac

BLENDS WITH
Bergamot, Lemongrass, Sandalwood, Patchouli, Orange, Mandarin

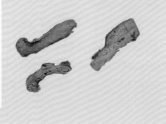

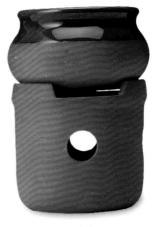

Vaporizing
The sweet scent of Ylang Ylang makes another good remedy for tension.

Carrier Oils Introduction

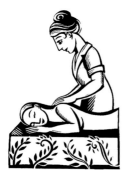

Facilitators
*Carrier oils are vegetable oils in which
the essential oils are diluted before being
massaged into the skin.*

What they are

To perform an aromatherapy massage,
the essential oils need to be diluted in a
vegetable oil, also called a "carrier" oil;
this allows the therapeutic properties of
the essential oils to be absorbed through
the skin surface. Many carrier oils are
crushed from nuts or seeds, from sources
like sweet almonds, grapeseeds, or
sunflower seeds. More exotic fatty oils are
obtained from the flesh of the avocado,
for example. Vegetable oils like these, as
well as the wonderful jojoba bean, which
yields a liquid wax, are very similar in
consistency to the skin's own natural oils,
and therefore give the skin suppleness,
a smooth texture, and a silky feel.

What to purchase

It is important to look for high quality
carrier oils, which can usually be found
in health food outlets or ordered from
specialist aromatherapy suppliers. Try to
buy cold-pressed carrier oils, preferably
as unrefined as possible, since this
preserves all the useful vitamins and
minerals. Some carrier oils have to
undergo a certain amount of processing,
but try to avoid supermarket vegetable
oils, which will have been chemically
treated. If you store your carrier oils in the
refrigerator, they should last up to nine
months. It is useful to note that petroleum
products like jelly or baby oil are not
recommended for use in aromatherapy,
because they are not well-absorbed by
the skin.

Other carrier products

Essential oils can also be dissolved in the
fat content of a cream or lotion. In specific
aromatherapy terms, creams and lotions
are both simple emulsifications of a

vegetable oil (such as, for example, sweet almond), with extra fat content—frequently something like cocoa butter or beeswax—and a floral water, for example rose. Later in this section you will find instructions for making your own cream or lotion base, or of course you can always buy this from specialist aromatherapy suppliers.

Creams are relatively heavy and give extra nourishment to the skin, while lotions usually have a more milky consistency and feel lighter on the skin. Again, it is best to avoid petroleum-based products—like aqueous cream or bases containing paraffin—since these are not compatible with the skin's own oils. Aromatherapy is most effective when it relies on high quality natural ingredients in order to achieve the best results.

SWEET ALMOND *Prunus dulcis, syn. P. amygdalus*

This extremely nutritious vegetable oil was used by the Romans in skincare preparations. It is native to the Middle East, and is now grown in the Mediterranean region. Used as a skin beautifier for hundreds of years, sweet almond oil is still used by the cosmetic industry in creams, lotions, and other skincare products. It is also one of the most popular carrier oils used in aromatherapy. The essential fatty acids in sweet almond oil play an important role in skin health, maintaining good circulation, and hair growth.

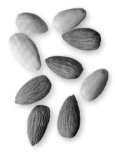

Datafile

BOTANICAL NAME
Prunus amygdalus dulcis

PLANT TYPE
Sweet almond tree

CARRIER OIL FROM
Pressed nuts, which yield about half their weight in vegetable oil

APPEARANCE & TEXTURE
Light yellow in color, rich and smooth to apply, leaving a silky feel to the skin

KEY INGREDIENTS
Good source of essential fatty acids

SAFETY NOTES
May not be tolerated by individuals allergic to nuts

KEEP FOR
6–9 months

RECOMMENDED USES
Protecting and nourishing the skin, as a massage base for dry and delicate skins

Beauty role
The oil from the Sweet Almond tree has long been used in skincare.

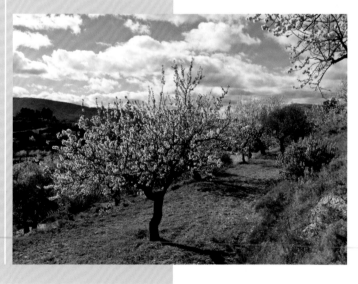

JOJOBA *Simmondsia chinensis*

This carrier product has a long history of use among the Native Americans of both Arizona and New Mexico, where the climate is very harsh. The difference between jojoba and other carriers is that it is a liquid wax rather than a vegetable oil; it works very well for facial care, because it resembles the skin's own natural oils. It also keeps well, and creates excellent skincare creams for all skin types, maintaining a healthy, supple complexion.

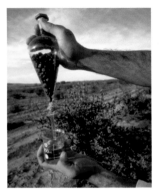

Datafile

BOTANICAL NAME
Simmondsia chinensis

PLANT TYPE
Jojoba bush, up to 1 meter (3 feet) in height, with small dark beans that contain the wax

CARRIER OIL FROM
Beans

APPEARANCE & TEXTURE
Golden, with a smooth texture, well-absorbed by all skin types

KEY INGREDIENTS
Liquid wax esters, similar to the skin's own oils

SAFETY NOTES
None

KEEP FOR
Up to 1 year

RECOMMENDED USES
Massage for all skin types. Jojoba combines with the skin's sebum to dissolve dirt and remove impurities. It makes a very good preservative for aromatherapy blends; try 25 percent jojoba to 75 percent grapeseed or sweet almond oils as a base, before adding your essential oils. On its own it is also a very good base for perfumes

Extraction
Jojoba wax is extracted from the beans of the bush.

Healthy appearance
Jojoba is an all-round skin and hair tonic.

Sweet Almond & Jojoba Blends

Sweet Almond Skin Treats

Sweet almond oil is a vitamin-E-rich carrier oil excellent for restoring the complexion and improving dry skin. The numbers next to the oils refer to the number of drops to be used.

TREATMENT	OILS	METHOD
Facial pamper	2 Neroli 3 Petitgrain 5 Orange in 4 teaspoons (20 milliliters) of sweet almond oil	Massage half a teaspoonful gently into the face at night
Sensitive skin balm	2 Rose 2 Sandalwood in 4 teaspoons (20 milliliters) of sweet almond oil	Apply half a teaspoonful to the affected area, especially in the evening
Sunburn rescue	4 Lavender 2 Peppermint 4 Palmarosa in 4 teaspoons (20 milliliters) of sweet almond oil	Apply half a teaspoonful to sore skin with very gentle strokes
Chapped hand nourishment	3 Geranium 5 Lavender 2 Neroli in 4 teaspoons (20 milliliters) of sweet almond oil	Apply half a teaspoonful to hands, especially after doing the dishes
Cracked heel balm	3 Frankincense 3 Patchouli 4 Lavender in 4 teaspoons (20 milliliters) of sweet almond oil	Apply half a teaspoonful to the affected area, especially at night

Jojoba Perfumes

Jojoba makes an excellent carrier for creating your own perfumes.
Dab a little behind the ears, on the wrists, or men might like to try a
little as an aftershave. The numbers next to the oils refer to the number
of drops to be used.

TREATMENT	OILS
Sensual perfume, to appeal to both men and women. A mysterious enchanting fragrance	2 Jasmine 3 Patchouli 5 Sandalwood in 4 teaspoons (20 milliliters) of jojoba oil
Euphoric perfume, to uplift the spirits, chase away the blues, and bring a sense of peace	5 Orange 2 Neroli 3 Frankincense in 4 teaspoons (20 milliliters) of jojoba oil
Earthing perfume, to bring you back to your center when it's all too much	5 Patchouli 3 Vetiver 2 Rose in 4 teaspoons (20 milliliters) of jojoba oil
Refreshing perfume, to waken your spirits, brighten your mood, give you energy and a positive boost	5 Lemon 3 Rosemary 2 Lemongrass in 4 teaspoons (20 milliliters) of jojoba oil
Fruity fragrance, to bring you a carefree sense of childhood freedom and zest	5 Orange 3 Mandarin 2 Benzoin in 4 teaspoons (20 milliliters) of jojoba oil

AVOCADO

Persea americana This carrier oil comes from the flesh of the avocado pear. First discovered in South America, the Aztecs were fond of the fruit, claiming it was an aphrodisiac. It was in use in Mexico in the 16th century as a tonic for illness. Nowadays, it is an important cosmetic ingredient, used in a range of products including bath oils, hair conditioners, and lipsticks. It has a smoothing effect on the upper skin layers.

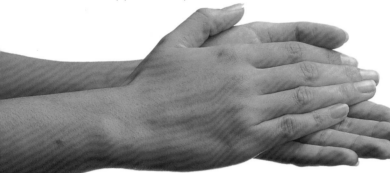

Conditioning
Avocado is a very rich conditioner of dry skin.

Datafile

BOTANICAL NAME
Persea americana

PLANT TYPE
Avocado tree

CARRIER OIL FROM
Ripe avocado pears

APPEARANCE & TEXTURE
If unrefined, avocado oil will have a deep green color and a very nutty fragrance. Refined oil is available, and has less useful nutrients and a paler color

KEY INGREDIENTS
Vitamins A and D, potassium, lecithin

SAFETY NOTES
None

KEEP FOR
6–9 months

RECOMMENDED USES
Soothing for eczema and very dry, chapped, or peeling skin

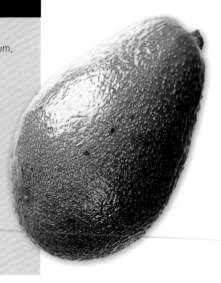

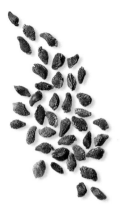

EVENING PRIMROSE *Oenothera biennis* Used as

a wound-healing ingredient by Native American medicine men, evening primrose oil is a star of natural medicine, prized as an internal tonic as well as for external use. It is rich in gamma linolenic acid (GLA), which is not present in the body, and has to be obtained from the diet in order to promote the formation of prostaglandins, which are essential to many activities in the body. Imbalances of prostaglandins lie behind many menstrual disorders in women.

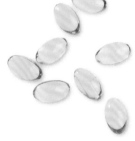

Datafile

BOTANICAL NAME
Oenothera biennis

PLANT TYPE
Tall herb with slender leaves and yellow flowers that bloom in the evenings

CARRIER OIL FROM
Flowers

APPEARANCE & TEXTURE
Light yellow in color, fairly sticky texture

KEY INGREDIENTS
High proportions of GLA

SAFETY NOTES
None

KEEP FOR
Up to one month if the oil is exposed to the air. It is best to buy large capsules of the oil from a drugstore, prick with a pin and squeeze the contents into your hand each time you want to use it

RECOMMENDED USES
Soothing for eczema and dry or damaged skin. Good for poor circulation and dandruff

Healing
Evening Primrose was used by Native Americans as a wound healer.

Avocado & Evening Primrose Blends

Avocado Nourishment Blends

Avocado is a particularly rich carrier oil, full of vitamins. The essential oils blended with it need to be quite powerful to mask its pronounced nutty odor. The following skin nourishing blends will feed extremely dry skin. The numbers next to the oils refer to the number of drops to be used.

TREATMENT	OILS	METHOD
Earthy and soothing	3 Vetiver 7 Sandalwood in 4 teaspoons (20 milliliters) of avocado oil	Apply half a teaspoonful to the affected area, morning and night
Skin healing for chapped skin	6 Frankincense 4 Roman Chamomile in 4 teaspoons (20 milliliters) of avocado oil	Apply half a teaspoonful to the affected area, morning and night
For sensitive skin	2 Rose 2 Neroli in 4 teaspoons (20 milliliters) of avocado oil	Apply half a teaspoonful to the affected area, morning and night
Skin balancing	3 Geranium 7 Orange in 4 teaspoons (20 milliliters) of avocado oil	Apply half a teaspoonful to the affected area, morning and night
Skin healing with tropical fragrance	6 Palmarosa 4 Patchouli in 4 teaspoons (20 milliliters) of avocado oil	Apply half a teaspoonful to the affected area, morning and night

Evening Primrose Skin Repair Blends

The gamma linolenic acid (GLA) in evening primrose oil is extremely important for treating skin damage, such as eczema or psoriasis. It is relatively expensive to buy; one of the best ways is to obtain 1,000 IU capsules from a drugstore, and prick them with a sterilized needle, squeezing the contents into a small cup. One capsule will be enough to treat an affected area. The numbers next to the oils refer to the number of drops to be used.

TREATMENT	OILS	METHOD
Eczema—child aged between three and ten	1 Roman Chamomile per evening primrose capsule	Apply to the affected area, especially at night
Eczema—adult	1 Rose 1 Patchouli per evening primrose capsule	Apply to the affected area, especially at night
Psoriasis—child aged between three and ten	1 Lavender per evening primrose capsule	Apply to the affected area, especially at night
Psoriasis—adult	1 Roman Chamomile 1 Sandalwood per evening primrose capsule	Apply to the affected area, especially at night
Dry, flaking skin	1 Neroli 1 Geranium per evening primrose capsule	Apply to the affected area, especially at night

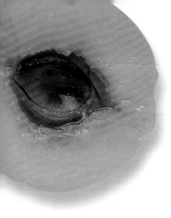

APRICOT KERNEL *Prunus armeniaca*

Prunus armeniaca The apricot tree is native to Armenia, but probably originated in China and Southeast Asia. It was introduced to England from Italy during the reign of King Henry VIII. Apricots are closely related to peaches and plums, and can be grown in cooler climates on a south-facing wall although in very cool weather they may not fruit. The oil is extracted from the stones of the fruit, and is a favorite in aromatherapy for facial massages.

Datafile

BOTANICAL NAME
Prunus armeniaca

PLANT TYPE
Hardy tree with white flowers tinged with red, ripening to a pale orange fruit

CARRIER OIL FROM
Kernels, which yield up to half their weight in oil

APPEARANCE & TEXTURE
Very light colored and light textured, nongreasy

KEY INGREDIENTS
Essential fatty acids

SAFETY NOTES
None

KEEP FOR
6–9 months

RECOMMENDED USES
Facial work on all skin types, including oily skins because it will not leave a greasy film

Trees
Apricot trees were first grown in England in Henry VIII's time.

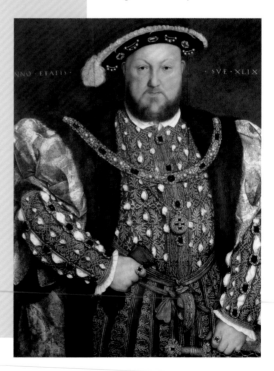

GRAPESEED

Vitis vinifera This carrier oil comes from the wine-producing regions of France, where it is extracted from grape pips. It is very popular as a massage oil in aromatherapy. It is nongreasy, leaving a pleasant feeling on the skin and little residue. It is also a useful alternative to sweet almond oil if you or anyone you are working on is allergic to nuts. It suits skins that are supple and do not need enriching.

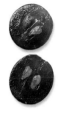

Versatility
Oil made from grapeseed suits all skin types.

Datafile

BOTANICAL NAME
Vitis vinifera

PLANT TYPE
Grapevine

CARRIER OIL FROM
Grapeseeds

APPEARANCE & TEXTURE
Very light green. Most grapeseed oil has been refined to a degree, because in its raw state it is unpalatable. It has no fragrance and a light texture

KEY INGREDIENTS
Polyunsaturated fatty acids

SAFETY NOTES
None

KEEP FOR
6–9 months

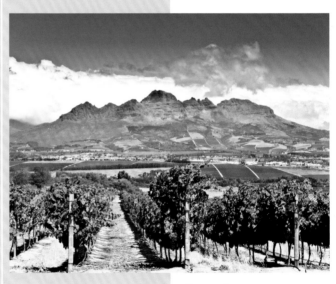

RECOMMENDED USES
Massage for all skin types, even oily

Extraction
Grapeseed oil is extracted from grape pips.

Apricot &
Grapeseed Blends

Apricot Kernel Facials

The light texture of apricot kernel oil makes it a very good choice for facial massage; it is easily absorbed by the skin. Here are some blends to try for special facial treats. The numbers next to the oils refer to the number of drops to be used. See pages 122–209 for massage tips and techniques.

TREATMENT	OILS	METHOD
Shaving oil for men, to help sore skin	4 Patchouli 6 Frankincense in 4 teaspoons (20 milliliters) of apricot kernel oil	Massage half a teaspoonful into the skin every day
Mature skin facial	3 Rose 7 Sandalwood in 4 teaspoons (20 milliliters) of apricot kernel oil	Massage half a teaspoonful into the skin, especially at night
Alternative mature skin facial	2 Jasmine 8 Orange in 4 teaspoons (20 milliliters) of apricot kernel oil	Massage half a teaspoonful into the skin, especially at night
Sensitive skin facial	2 Roman Chamomile 2 Palmarosa in 4 teaspoons (20 milliliters) of apricot kernel oil	Massage half a teaspoonful into the skin, especially at night
Teenage facial	4 Geranium 6 Lemon in 4 teaspoons (20 milliliters) of apricot kernel oil	Massage half a teaspoonful into the skin, especially at night

Grapeseed Body Blends

The light and nongreasy texture of grapeseed oil makes it the ideal carrier for skins that are well-lubricated already—it leaves a superb silky feel to the skin with no tackiness. The numbers next to the oils refer to the number of drops to be used. See pages 122–209 for massage tips and techniques.

TREATMENT	OILS	METHOD
Exotic blend, with a floral and citrus lift	3 Ylang Ylang 8 Bergamot in 4 teaspoons (20 milliliters) of grapeseed oil	Massage over the whole body
Oriental blend, earthy and woody, deeply relaxing for men and women	3 Patchouli 7 Sandalwood in 4 teaspoons (20 milliliters) of grapeseed oil	Massage over the whole body
Green blend, grassy, soft, and soothing with a hint of citrus	3 Clary Sage 7 Petitgrain in 4 teaspoons (20 milliliters) of grapeseed oil	Massage over the whole body
Citrus blend, total fruit immersion	5 Mandarin 5 Orange in 4 teaspoons (20 milliliters) of grapeseed oil	Massage over the whole body
Spicy blend to warm the skin	3 Ginger 7 Lemon in 4 teaspoons (20 milliliters) of grapeseed oil	Massage over the whole body

SUNFLOWER *Helianthus annus*

Originally from Mexico and Peru, the sunflower can grow up to 11⅓ feet (3.5 meters) in height. It was an important motif in the decoration of Aztec temples, where the sun was worshiped. It is a productive plant, because as well as harvesting the seeds, the stalks can be used in papermaking. Sunflower oil is extracted from fully ripened seeds, which contain about 40 percent oil.

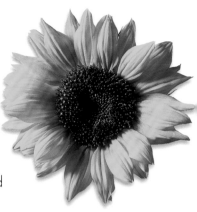

Sun worship
The Aztecs adorned many of their temples with sunflower symbols.

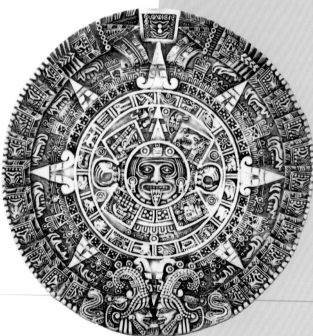

Datafile

BOTANICAL NAME
Helianthus annus

PLANT TYPE
Tall flower with large, circular seedhead

CARRIER OIL FROM
Pressed seeds

APPEARANCE & TEXTURE
Light golden color, light texture

KEY INGREDIENTS
High levels of vitamin E, polyunsaturated fatty acids

SAFETY NOTES
None

KEEP FOR
6–9 months

RECOMMENDED USES
Massage for all skin types, useful for mature skins due to the vitamin E content

WHEAT GERM *Triticum durum* Wheat has been grown for over 10,000 years, and wheat-germ oil has been found in Egyptian tombs dating back 2,000 years. The oil is extracted from the germ of the wheat, which contains many vitamins and minerals. Wheat-germ oil is an extremely rich source of skin-nourishing ingredients, useful for treating dry or mature complexions, and also acts as a natural preservative for aromatherapy blends. It is rich in vitamin E, which is a natural antioxidant.

Datafile

BOTANICAL NAME
Triticum durum

PLANT TYPE
Cereal grain

CARRIER OIL FROM
Germ of wheat

APPEARANCE & TEXTURE
Orange-brown color, thick consistency, bitter smell. Best used as an enriching carrier added to a lighter oil such as sunflower, try 20 percent wheat germ to 80 percent lighter oil.

KEY INGREDIENTS
High levels of vitamin E, essential fatty acids

SAFETY NOTES
None

KEEP FOR
Up to 1 year

Extraction
The rich oil derived from wheat comes from the germ of the plant.

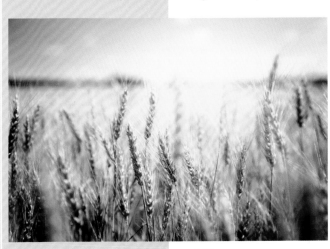

RECOMMENDED USES
Massage for very dry, mature skin, good for eczema and psoriasis

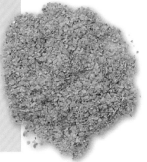

Sunflower & Wheat-germ Blends

Sunflower is a light-textured carrier oil, rich in vitamins, that leaves a silky feel on the skin. Use these blends to nourish your skin at times when it is more exposed to the elements. The numbers next to the oils refer to the number of drops to be used.

TREATMENT	OILS	METHOD
Cooling blend, soft and gently minty	7 Roman Chamomile 3 Peppermint in 4 teaspoons (20 milliliters) of sunflower oil	Apply half a teaspoonful to the affected areas. Best applied at night
Refreshing blend, with a hint of cologne	5 Lavender 5 Petitgrain in 4 teaspoons (20 milliliters) of sunflower oil	Apply half a teaspoonful to the affected areas. Best applied at night
Soothing blend, rosy soft	6 Palmarosa 4 Geranium in 4 teaspoons (20 milliliters) of sunflower oil	Apply half a teaspoonful to the affected areas. Best applied at night
Calming blend, vanilla-like and fruity	2 Benzoin 8 Orange in 4 teaspoons (20 milliliters) of sunflower oil	Apply half a teaspoonful to the affected areas. Best applied at night
Balancing blend, herbal and green	4 Clary Sage 6 Sweet Marjoram in 4 teaspoons (20 milliliters) of sunflower oil	Apply half a teaspoonful to the affected areas. Best applied at night

Wheat-germ Antioxidant Facials

Wheat-germ carrier oil is extremely useful as an antioxidant because it is rich in vitamin E. It can be very helpful for toning and reviving the facial area. It has quite a strong, slightly bitter scent and is tacky to use on its own, so it is best to make a carrier oil mixture of 1 teaspoon (5 milliliters) of wheat-germ oil to 3 teaspoons (15 milliliters) of apricot kernel oil. The numbers next to the oils refer to the number of drops to be used. See pages 122–209 for massage tips and techniques.

CONDITION	OILS	METHOD
Dry skin blend, floral and uplifting, using good skin tonic oils	3 Neroli 7 Frankincense in a carrier oil mixture (see above)	Massage half a teaspoonful well into the face, especially at night
Mature skin blend, with a woody, floral scent, and nourishing to the skin	3 Rose 7 Sandalwood in a carrier oil mixture (see above)	Massage half a teaspoonful well into the face, especially at night
Combination skin blend, with a floral, soothing scent, good for balancing the skin	4 Geranium 6 Lemon in a carrier oil mixture (see above)	Massage half a teaspoonful well into the face, especially at night
Oily skin blend, toning and astringent, encourages cleansing	3 Juniper 7 Cypress in a carrier oil mixture (see above)	Massage half a teaspoonful well into the face, especially at night
Sensitive skin blend, woody and light, very gentle	2 Patchouli 2 Lavender in a carrier oil mixture (see above)	Massage half a teaspoonful well into the face, especially at night

BASE CREAM

A base cream delivers essential oils very specifically to an area; it also nourishes the skin without leaving a residue. A base cream contains a combination of vegetable oils blended with a flower water, such as rose water, and emulsified with beeswax to stabilize it. You can buy unfragranced cream, but check that the ingredients are plant-based.

1 *Put the beeswax and sweet almond oil in a glass dish. Heat over simmering water in a deep-sided pot, stirring gently, until the mixture goes clear and reaches 140°F (60°C). At the same time, put the rosewater in the other glass dish, and heat over simmering water to the same temperature.*

2 *Remove both dishes from the heat, and slowly add the rosewater to the oil mixture, drop by drop, whisking constantly.*

3 *When all the water is used up, add up to 30 drops combination of your chosen essential oils. Stir in, pour the cream into the jar, and refrigerate; it will then set. This cream will have a shelf life of up to 3 weeks.*

Making Your Own Cream

Makes about 12 teaspoons (60 grams)

2 teaspoons (10 grams) beeswax

4 teaspoons (20 milliliters) sweet almond oil

4 teaspoons (20 milliliters) rose water

You will also need two deep-sided pots, two heat-resistant glass dishes to sit over the pots like double boilers, a whisk, a food thermometer, and a 2-ounce (60-gram) amber glass jar, available from a pharmacy.

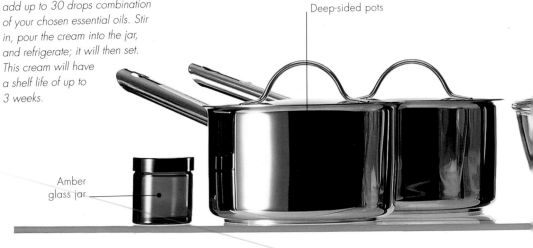

Deep-sided pots

Amber glass jar

BASE LOTION

This lotion is a more liquid version of a cream, with a milkier consistency. It is lighter on the skin but still nourishing, and leaves a soft feel. It is possible to buy unfragranced lotion or cream from the chemist or an essential oil supplier; however, again, you should check that there are no animal or petroleum-derived ingredients in these products.

Making Your Own Lotion

Makes about 4 tablespoons (60 milliliters)

3 teaspoons (15 grams) beeswax

4 teaspoons (20 milliliters) jojoba oil

6 teaspoons (30 milliliters) rosewater

You will also need two deep-sided pots, two heat-resistant glass dishes to sit over the pots like double boilers, a whisk, a food thermometer, and a ¼ pint (100 milliliters) amber glass bottle, available from a pharmacy.

1 In one glass dish, heat the beeswax and jojoba oil over simmering water until they combine and reach 140°F (60°C). At the same time, in the other glass dish, heat the rosewater over simmering water to the same temperature.

2 Remove both dishes from the heat. Add the rosewater to the oil mixture drop by drop, whisking continuously.

3 Add up to 30 drops of a combination of your chosen oils. Stir in, pour the lotion into the bottle, and refrigerate. The lotion will have a shelf life of about 3–4 weeks.

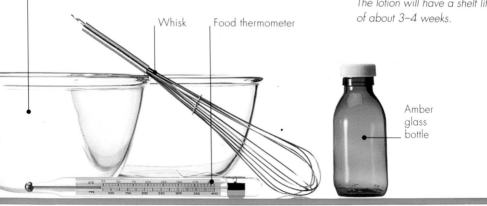

Heat-resistant glass dish

Whisk   Food thermometer

Amber glass bottle

Base Cream &
Base Lotion Blends

Base Cream Blends

The higher fat content in a cream makes it good to apply to specific problem areas. Base cream is also very useful for general skin care. Measure your cream into a pot, add the oils, and stir with a small spoon. The numbers next to the oils refer to the number of drops to be used.

TREATMENT	OILS	METHOD
First aid cream, very useful to keep in the medicine cabinet	5 Lavender 5 Tea Tree in 4 teaspoons (20 grams) of base cream	Apply when necessary
Skin repair cream, for deep cuts and abrasions	5 Roman Chamomile in 4 teaspoons (20 grams) of base cream	Apply when necessary
Super hand cream, for general hand care	3 Neroli 7 Geranium in 4 teaspoons (20 grams) of base cream	Work cream into the hands when necessary, especially after doing the washing up
Foot care cream, for aching and cold feet	4 Peppermint 6 Black Pepper in 4 teaspoons (20 grams) of base cream	Apply when necessary
Nail care cream, for cracked and split nails	4 Rose 6 Atlas Cedarwood in 4 teaspoons (20 grams) of base cream	Apply to the affected area

Base Lotion Blends

Base lotion can be used as an alternative to carrier oil, particularly for facial blends where an oily residue is undesirable. Measure the lotion into a bottle or jar and add the oils, stirring or shaking them together.

TREATMENT	OILS	METHOD
Combination skin blend, for balancing	4 Neroli 6 Geranium in 4 teaspoons (20 milliliters) of base lotion	Massage into the skin
Oily skin blend, toning and soothing	6 Lavender 4 Lemon in 4 teaspoons (20 milliliters) of base lotion	Massage into the skin
Acne blend, good for infected spots	3 Juniper 7 Tea Tree in 4 teaspoons (20 milliliters) of base lotion	Apply to the affected area
Acne blend, good if skin is dry in patches	4 Geranium 6 Lavender in 4 teaspoons (20 milliliters) of base lotion	Apply to the affected area
Shaving blend, skin soothing, for face and legs	5 Sandalwood 5 Patchouli in 4 teaspoons (20 milliliters) of base lotion	Massage into the affected area

PRACTICAL AROMATHERAPY

In this section you will find plenty of information about how to go about consulting a professional aromatherapist, as well as a complete aromatherapy treatment for you to follow, with step-by-step instructions for massaging the back, feet and legs, arms and hands, abdomen, neck and shoulders, and face. With plenty of oils to choose from and the many blends suggested in this book, all you now need to try out some aromatherapy is a willing volunteer. As a general guide, try to work on simple things to begin with—aches and pains or stiff backs and shoulders are a good place to start. If you are a beginner, keep to the techniques advised here and be very gentle on any painful areas. The application of aromatherapy can be pleasant and fulfilling to offer to family and friends.

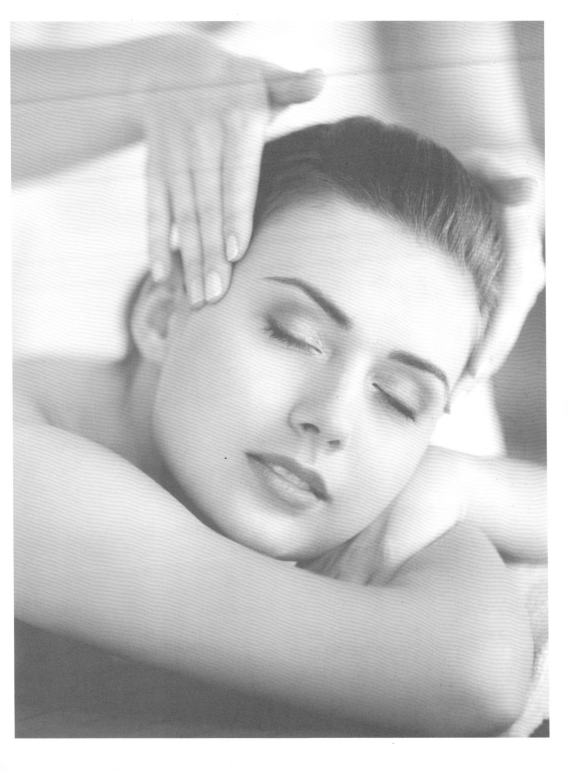

Consulting a Professional: A Typical Session

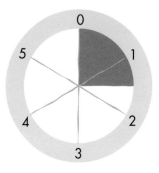

Treatment

A treatment often lasts for 1½ hours.

While it is pleasant to use aromatherapy techniques on yourself, there is no substitute for a visit to a professional practitioner. Below is a general idea of what you can expect from a visit to a trained aromatherapist, someone who has a thorough knowledge of what he or she is using, and who blends essential oils specifically to suit your needs. It is useful to ask therapists about their training, how long they have been practicing, as well as checking their membership of a professional body.

Consultation

Before deciding which blend to use, your therapist will spend some time with you, discussing details of your medical background, any current conditions you may be receiving treatment for, any allergies you may have, any other issues that have a bearing on safety—pregnancy, for example—as well as any emotional stresses you may be experiencing. From this very detailed information, the therapist will agree the focus of the treatment with you, then three or four essential oils will be chosen to help with your physical and emotional symptoms. It is important that your therapist lets you smell the oils for your blend first, to ensure you will be happy with the end result—you will relax more deeply if you like the fragrance.

Treatment

You will be asked to undress and will then be wrapped in a towel. At all times you are covered by towels and kept warm; only the area that is being massaged will actually be undraped. The therapist will tell you in what order you can expect to receive the massage, and will already have blended the essential oils in a carrier oil, which is then applied to your skin. It is important that you tell your therapist if you feel uncomfortable at any time during the treatment, although generally you will just want to relax into the experience and enjoy it. You will be left to rest for a few moments at the end of the session before getting dressed again. Aromatherapy treatment is holistic, working on many different levels. Sometimes the benefits will be felt quickly, but at other times patience is needed, particularly if your problem is a chronic one.

Key Essential Oil

Mandarin, like all citrus oils, is very popular as a destressor and can encourage a positive mood.

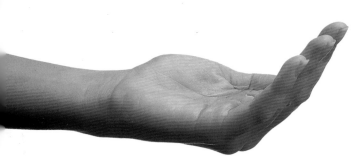

Massage oil
Pour a little of your blend into the palm of your hand.

BACK MASSAGE: EFFLEURAGE

The back is a good area to work on, especially if you or your friend are new to massaging. It is a large expanse of skin that responds very quickly to touch, and allows techniques to be practiced easily. Effleurage, the first stage of back massage, consists of a series of gentle soothing stokes, using your whole hand.

1 *Working up from the lower back, with a hand on either side of the spine, glide up and fan out over the shoulders. Then glide the hands back down the sides to begin again. Repeat at least six times. Build up to a rhythm.*

2 *Starting from the lower back, with the heels of the hands on either side of the spine, fingers pointing out to the side, fan the hands out in a small circle and return to the starting point. Carry out three strokes over the lower back, three over the mid-back, and three over the shoulders.*

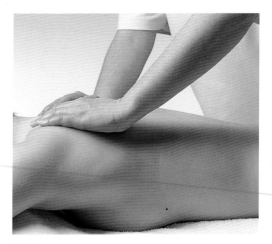

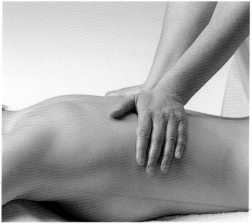

Warming the Back

The pressure in these soothing strokes should be firm but light; they are designed to warm and ease out the back in preparation for the deeper work to come. It is very important that you start the routine in this way, with warming strokes, otherwise the massage could feel very uncomfortable or even painful.

3 *With both hands on the person's left lower back area, make a long, figure-eight shape all the way up from the lower back to the shoulders, then repeat gently over the spine, and then over the right side.*

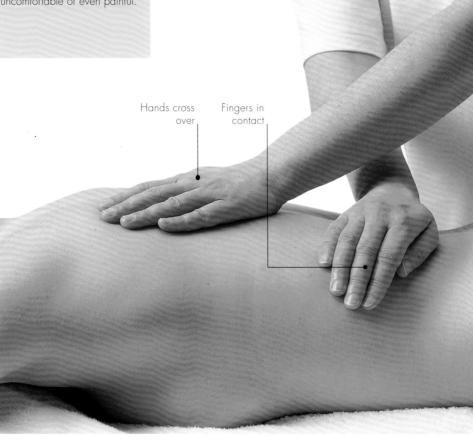

Hands cross over

Fingers in contact

Back Massage: A Key Treatment for Health

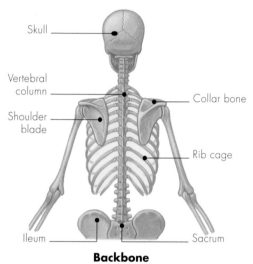

Skull

Vertebral column

Shoulder blade

Collar bone

Rib cage

Ileum

Sacrum

Backbone

The back is a complex structure.

The back is a very complex structure, vital to the upright way that we walk, with nerves fanning out from every vertebra connecting it to every part of the body. Poor posture, incorrect seating, even the wrong shoes can affect the state of the back. Every bone counterbalances every other bone, allowing an extensive range of movement, but it is quickly put off-balance or injured if a heavy load is lifted wrongly, or long periods are spent in a cramped position—when gardening, for example.

Muscle massage

Muscles are linked to the bony frame of the back, and pain in them is often the first sign of a possible back problem. Massage works to ease out pain or cramping in the muscles, allowing free movement. If the pain returns, then there may be a structural problem underlying the muscle tissue, which needs treatment by an osteopath or chiropractor.

Essential back oils

Essential oils for aches and pains are added to massage blends. They warm and increase the circulation to the area that is being treated, helping to dispose of any toxins trapped in the muscle fibers. Ginger is particularly good, as well as Lemongrass or Rosemary, all of which have strong penetrating fragrances as well as a zesty effect on the muscles.

The back feels tingly and energized after being massaged with these oils. For evening massage it is good to choose oils that are more relaxing in fragrance but that are still good for releasing tension; Vetiver, Lavender, or Sweet Marjoram are very useful in this instance, being deeply soothing to smell but also useful as pain-relieving, warming oils.

It is important to start your back massage with long, flowing strokes that warm the whole area, before attempting to carry out any deeper work. This relaxes your friend, releases any tension that has accumulated in the muscles, and warms your hands too. Just simple strokes can calm a person down if he or she is feeling either stressed or anxious.

Key Essential Oil

Vetiver has a deeply warming effect on tight muscles and can be used to help backache.

BACK MASSAGE: KNEADING

Moving on to a series of deeper strokes, here we use the hands to apply a wringing pressure to large areas of muscle tissue. The movement is a bit like making bread: one hand follows the other, squeezing out the muscle each time to ease tension in the tissue. Kneading may take a little practice to master; try the movement out on a soft cushion first. Check with your friend that you are not pinching, which can feel uncomfortable. Slow work is very relaxing to receive, quicker kneading is more invigorating.

1 *Pick up and knead the large muscles on either side of the shoulders—the trapezius muscles—which really respond well to kneading. You can do this with one hand each side, or two hands together. Knead for a few minutes.*

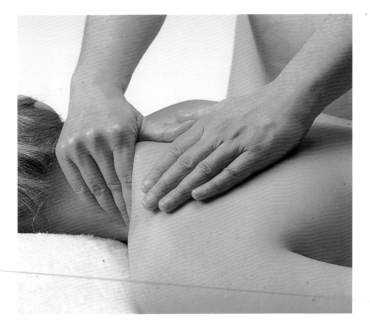

2 Now knead all the way down the side of the body, with firm, not ticklish, pressure. Work over to the other side and back up to the shoulders. Repeat this sequence twice.

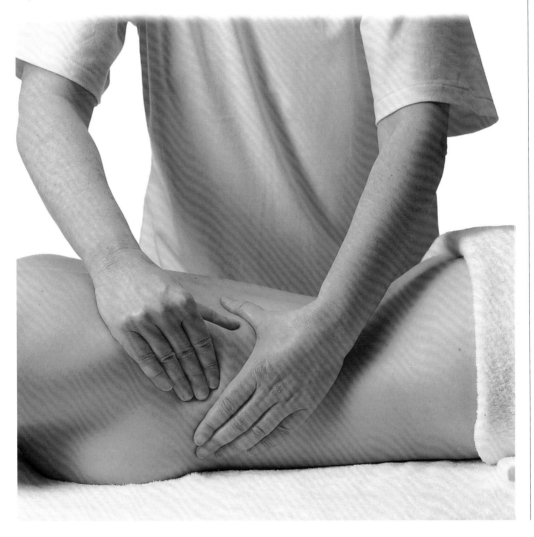

Reading the Back

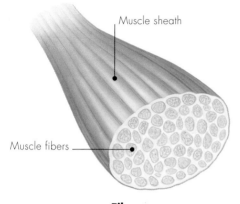

Muscle sheath

Muscle fibers

Fibers
*Muscle fibers are
arranged in bundles
within a sheath.*

As you massage the back, your hands are working on the soft tissue, the muscles under the skin. Muscle tissue is made up of fibers. When they contract, they use up oxygen and glucose to provide energy. These fibers give off waste products, such as lactic acid and carbon dioxide, which are normally carried away by the blood and lymphatic systems. However, build-up of these waste products causes pain and stiffness. Massage increases blood supply to the painful area so the waste products can be removed.

Evaluating problems

You may feel a number of things as you massage a friend's back. Areas of cold skin are due to poor circulation and need careful work in order to warm up the tissue. Essential oils such as Black Pepper are very helpful in such circumstances, adding to the warming nature of the massage.

Areas that feel stiff and that do not move easily could be because of a build-up of waste products or something more long-term, such as an injury or arthritis. Check the cause with your friend. As a general rule, please be very careful when working on an area with limited available movement; if you are in any doubt it is better to leave it alone.

Grittiness or small lumps in the muscle fibers that ease out as you work may be nodules of lactic acid build-up. As you work, with kneading or pressure (see pages 130–31), you may well feel them ease away. Keep checking with your friend that the pressure is feeling comfortable.

Any doubts?

If you find any unusual lumps on the body while you are treating somebody, it is best to leave them alone and to refer your friend to his or her doctor. As a rule, massage is wonderfully beneficial; however, it always pays to be careful and to observe what is happening as you massage the body and feel the way it responds.

When not to massage

A massage is generally a useful treatment. However, do not work on the body if your friend feels at all unwell.

If they have a known medical condition, such as high blood pressure, varicose veins, or arthritis, you should keep the massage very light and they should consult a doctor or a professional therapist before undergoing more treatment of this kind.

Key Essential Oil

Juniper is a powerful cleanser and helps detoxify the tissues.

BACK MASSAGE: PRESSURE WORK

The pressure in this particular massage technique is applied using mainly the thumbs, leaning into the movement with all your bodyweight. Apply the pressure gradually, since your thumbs need to get used to performing this activity, and check with your friend that the intensity of the pressure is comfortable. A certain level of pain may be experienced if the area is at all stiff, but it should not be unbearable. Stroke the area in order to release the pressure afterward.

1 *Gently position your friend's arm across the back at a level the person is comfortable with. This presents the shoulder blade to you.*

2 *Supporting under the shoulder with one hand, use the thumb of the other hand to apply a triangle of small pressures all around the shoulder blade. Release the arm gently then repeat on the other arm. This work really helps stiff shoulders.*

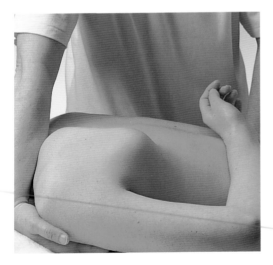

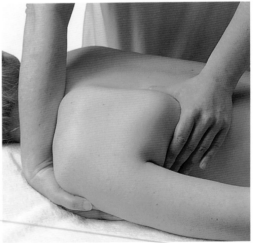

3 With thumbs in the ridges on either side of the spine, apply a series of thumb pressures for around 10 seconds each time, all the way up to the shoulders. Do this twice. Check that the amount of pressure is comfortable for your friend.

4 At the base of the spine there is a large bony area called the sacrum. Apply a triangle of pressures to this area, coming gradually inward, toward the tailbone.

5 Repeat the sequence from the beginning, only now with more pressure. Building up a steady rhythm, repeat several times. Your hands will feel really warm.

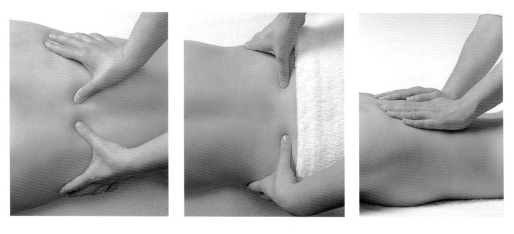

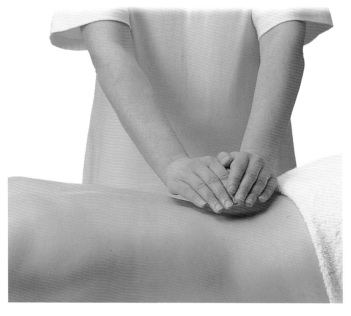

6 Cup the hands over the base of the spine and hold them there until you feel heat gather. Slowly lift the hands away—this can give your friend a sensation like floating.

Pressure Work: How to Use It

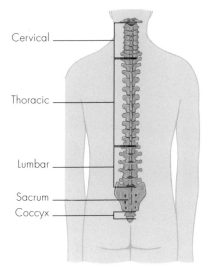

Cervical

Thoracic

Lumbar

Sacrum

Coccyx

Back divisions

The spine is divided into five areas.

Eastern cultures, such as the Japanese and Chinese, have ancient traditions involving the use of finger pressures in massage. In Japan, this massage is called *shiatsu*, and involves applying pressure to specific areas in order to regulate and restore the flow of the life force, or *chi*, through channels called meridians. This in turn promotes the healing of different areas of the body, relieves pain, and restores energy. To become proficient in shiatsu takes many years of dedicated study; however, some of the pressure points are easily accessed for simple, day-to-day use.

Everyday shiatsu

The pressure points along the spine are interesting because they link to all the major body systems: on the upper spine they help lung congestion; on the mid-back, digestive problems; and on the lower back, the reproductive organs and the process of elimination. The triangle of points in the area of the sacrum at the base of the spine is very useful for period pain and lower back pain. You need to apply pressure gently, slowly building up to a tolerable level for your friend. When you reach that level, hold it for about 5 seconds. You can then release the area by circle stroking it gently to ease any stiffness.

Incorporating pressure work

In aromatherapy massage it helps to incorporate pressure point work into your routine to add to the benefit of the general massage strokes; this way you can help relieve pain and work on very specific areas. If you find a point is very painful for your friend, try applying 1 drop Lavender onto that area and repeating the pressure. It is normal to warm the whole area first with sweeping strokes, then ease out any tension using kneading, followed by pressure work. If you try to apply pressure too soon, your friend will tense up, making the process uncomfortable for both of you.

Remember the sequence

Warming, kneading, then pressure, followed by soothing strokes to finish, is the method you should always follow with aromatherapy massage. A good back massage is a wonderful, magical treatment, bringing deep relaxation.

FOOT MASSAGE: STRETCH

Your feet will walk you to the moon and back in a lifetime, so they say, and precious little thanks do they ever get for all the work they do for you. A foot massage is a perfect way to give your feet the attention they deserve. This first part of the foot massage routine really works on the feet to ease tension, while also warming and stretching them out. Cold feet are commonly linked to poor circulation. If your friend suffers from this problem, try rubbing the feet briskly before you start the massage. Speeding up the strokes shown here will also help to warm up cold feet.

1 *Hold the feet under both ankles, supporting them firmly but gently. Ask your friend to take a few slow, deep breaths.*

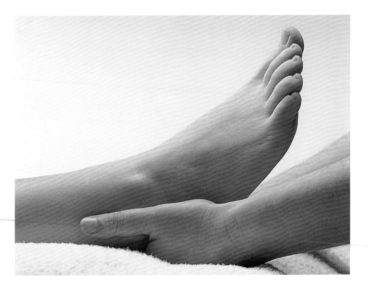

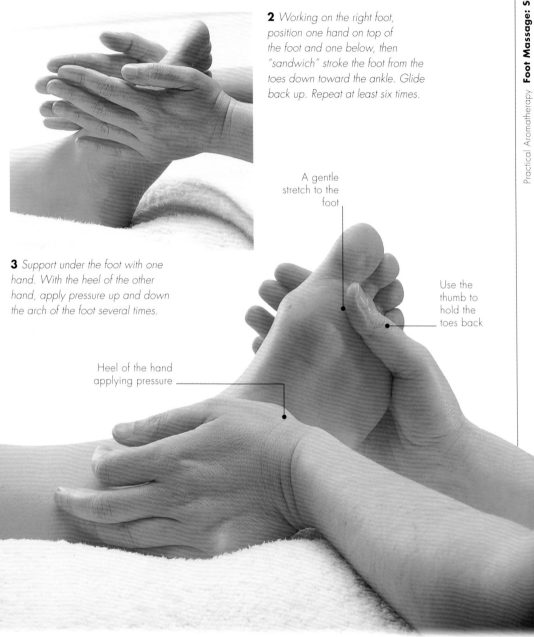

2 *Working on the right foot, position one hand on top of the foot and one below, then "sandwich" stroke the foot from the toes down toward the ankle. Glide back up. Repeat at least six times.*

3 *Support under the foot with one hand. With the heel of the other hand, apply pressure up and down the arch of the foot several times.*

A gentle
stretch to the
foot

Use the
thumb to
hold the
toes back

Heel of the hand
applying pressure

The Practice & Benefits of a Foot Massage

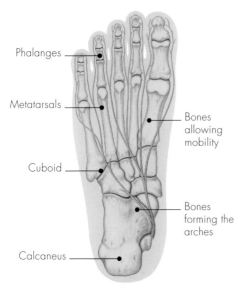

Foot structure
The foot is a complex area of human anatomy.

Phalanges

Metatarsals

Cuboid

Calcaneus

Bones allowing mobility

Bones forming the arches

The structure of the feet is amazing; almost a quarter of the bones in the whole body are to be found there. Bones, muscles, and ligaments are woven together in a piece of evolutionary engineering that provides a balanced framework to carry the weight of the whole person. The feet are able to eliminate waste products from the body in the form of sweat; strong foot odor can be a sign of toxin build-up within the system, as well as a sign of poor hygiene.

Begin clean

It is useful to cleanse the feet before working on them, using a footbath. This can greatly enhance the penetration of essential oils through the thicker skin layers once you begin massaging, as the damp skin allows for better absorption of the aromatherapy blend.

Treat the feet, treat the body

There are thousands of nerve endings in the feet that connect to the whole body. For that reason, a foot massage is very beneficial. By massaging the feet you are in effect treating the whole body; systems like reflexology work on exactly this basis. Essential oil blends are very beneficial here: using oils such as Rosemary to boost the circulation, or Neroli to calm nervous stress, a foot massage can be physically or psychologically useful. The feet are our connection to the Earth.

Very cold, numb feet can be a sign of being "disconnected," or not "grounded." Vetiver essential oil is very useful in a massage in this situation; it has a strong fragrance of earth and is very warming to the circulation. Just holding the foot for a few moment at the end of the massage is very calming.

Touch sensitive

A word about being ticklish. It is important to hold the foot steady as you work, and to keep the pressure gentle but firm. Strong strokes using the heel of the hand really help to instill confidence in your massage, and should also help if there is any oversensitivity to touch.

Key Essential Oil

Peppermint essential oil is wonderfully cooling to tired feet.

FOOT MASSAGE: UPPER FOOT

After a nice deep stretch, work on the upper part of the foot, where tendons and ligaments sit over the bones. The movements here are precise, but try not to press too hard, which can be uncomfortable for your friend. It is good to finish your foot massage with more sandwich strokes (see page 135) and glide off, before repeating on the other foot.

1 *With both hands on one foot, fingers laced above the foot, thumbs together underneath the middle toe, press all the way down the foot in a firm line, stretching all the bones as you go. Repeat twice.*

2 *Knead each toe between your fingers and give a gentle pull to stretch each one.*

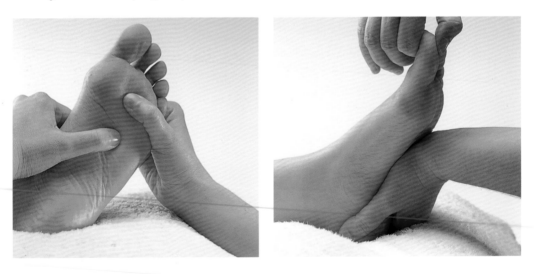

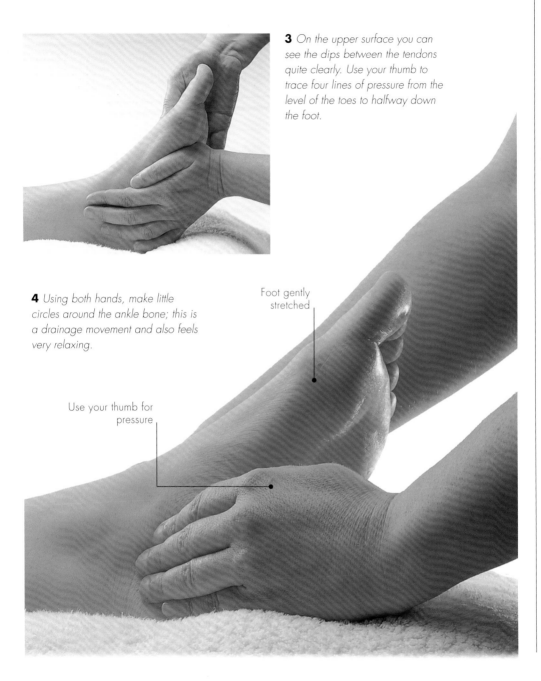

3 *On the upper surface you can see the dips between the tendons quite clearly. Use your thumb to trace four lines of pressure from the level of the toes to halfway down the foot.*

4 *Using both hands, make little circles around the ankle bone; this is a drainage movement and also feels very relaxing.*

Foot gently stretched

Use your thumb for pressure

Case Study: Bad Circulation

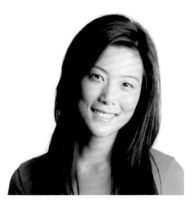

Lifestyle
*Janet needs to consider her lifestyle
as well as receive treatments.*

Consultation

Janet has come along for a treatment complaining of really cold feet. It is the middle of the hottest time of the year, so we are not linking it to the weather. She is surprised that it still bothers her at this time. She has a history of low blood pressure, which can be linked to cold extremities, and often feels lethargic and low in energy. She wants to be energized for her forthcoming vacation. When

asked about her routine, she says she sits in an office all day and has little time for any exercise after commuting home at night and looking after her husband and two children.

Treatment

As her therapist, I explain that we can use essential oils and massage to help her circulation, but she is going to need to do some work on this at home to make long-term improvements. I select a fresh, warming, and stimulating blend of 2 drops Lemongrass, 5 drops Black Pepper, and 3 drops Ginger in 4 teaspoons (20 milliliters) of sweet almond oil, and apply this in a full body massage, paying special attention to her feet and legs with kneading, cupping, and pressure work. A heat pad under her feet helps to keep them warm during the session. She relaxes very deeply and almost goes to sleep.

Self-care

I make up 8 teaspoons (40 milliliters) of the same blend of oils and suggest a personal routine each morning. First, Janet must use a skin-brush on her dry feet to stimulate the circulation, followed by a hot shower, then a simple massage of half a teaspoonful of the blend into her feet and lower legs. Her diet needs to include warming ingredients such as fresh ginger and chilies, and she needs to try to walk for 20 minutes each day.

Timescale

It will take around five weekly 90-minute sessions and a month of exercise and home massage to improve Janet's circulation. Often it takes teamwork to achieve results.

Key Essential Oil

Black Pepper essential oil has a warming effect and is a powerful circulation stimulant.

LEG MASSAGE: WARM UP

After a foot massage, this leg routine can be done with your friend still lying on their back, with no need for them to turn over. A leg massage really helps to soothe away tiredness, aches, and pains. When performing a leg massage, the pressure should always be worked upward, toward the heart, followed by gliding off as you come back, in order to encourage the circulation. Watch out for any bruises or varicose veins and ensure that you do not massage over these. One point worth making about treating men—make sure that you use plenty of the massage blend on your hands if the legs are very hairy, or it will feel uncomfortable to receive the massage.

1 *Start at the ankle, with both hands together. Stroke all the way up to the thigh and glide back. Repeat four times.*

2 *Support the knee with one hand, and use the heel of the other hand to knuckle the calf muscle.*

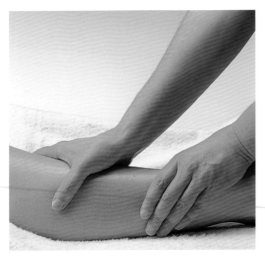

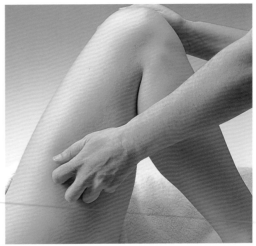

Fingertips working

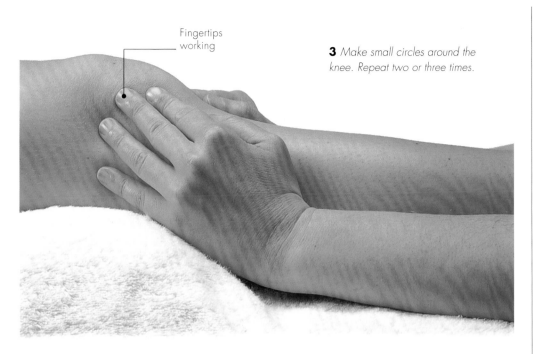

3 *Make small circles around the knee. Repeat two or three times.*

4 *Move up to the side of the leg and knead the upper thigh using a sideways movement.*

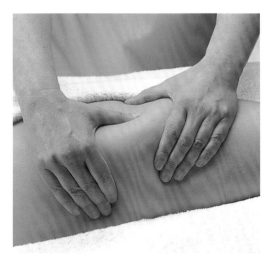

5 *Crisscross the hands over the thigh to really work the muscle. Repeat four times.*

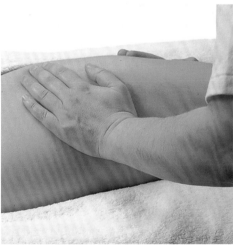

Leg Massage & Lymphatic Drainage

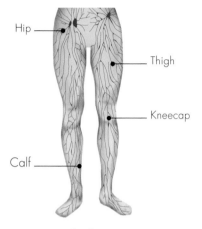

Hip

Thigh

Kneecap

Calf

The legs
*Poor diet and lack of exercise
can affect the legs.*

The legs have a tendency to feel the effects of a modern lifestyle. Too much sitting, not enough exercise, and high levels of toxins in our food can create waterlogged, fatty tissue in the thighs and also cause puffiness and water retention in the lower legs. An obsession with "orange-peel" skin (cellulite) can never be fully solved with external treatments; the attention to internal cleansing is extremely important, although often neglected.

A good diet

Aromatherapy is a holistic approach, where massage and essential oils will be given along with simple advice to improve lifestyle habits that may be impacting on health. Reducing the intake of salt and caffeine, as well as cutting out cigarettes and junk food, substituting wholefoods, springwater, and fresh juices like carrot or celery will be important parts of a treatment for fatty tissue and water retention in the legs.

Improving lymphatic drainage

There are specific massage techniques taught to professionals that can improve lymphatic drainage; the techniques illustrated in this book will assist that process, especially if the pressure is applied in an upward direction, toward the heart. Essential oils that particularly help fluid retention and cellulite are Juniper, Lemon, and Fennel, which can be combined at 3 drops each in 4 teaspoons (20 milliliters) of carrier oil,

and then massaged into the legs daily.
It is also helpful to take two baths each
week containing a teacup full of Epsom
salts, in order to increase the circulation
and elimination, and to try skin-brushing
before a bath or shower, followed by
application of a detoxifying blend.

Massage techniques

When massaging the legs, be careful not
to apply heavy pressure on the shins or
the kneecaps, instead keep the movement
light but firm. Any areas that are swollen
or puffy can have an aromatherapy blend
gently stroked on, but no heavy pressure
should be applied there. Any unusual
swelling should be referred to the doctor. It
also helps to raise the legs after treatment.

Key Essential Oil

Fennel essential oil is a very useful cleanser and
general detoxifier.

LEG MASSAGE: BUILDING PRESSURE

At this stage the leg needs to be bent upward and the foot placed flat on the couch or floor. If necessary you can sit gently on the foot in order to hold the leg steady and prevent it rocking from side to side. After these slow strokes, release the leg again so that once more it lies flat on the surface. Finish the massage routine with gentle stroking movements, and then repeat the whole routine on the other leg.

1 *With the leg bent, knead the calf muscles really thoroughly. You can also tap the calf with half-cupped hands to stimulate the circulation.*

2 *Making loose fists, knuckle under the thighs making lots of little circles with your fingers. Then set the leg back down.*

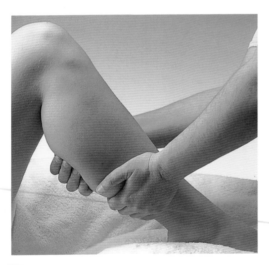

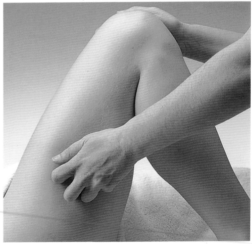

3 *Starting at the ankle, stroke up the leg, applying more pressure and increasing the speed. Repeat five to six times.*

4 *Starting at the ankle, make little, alternate flicking movements all the way up the leg and glide back. Repeat twice.*

5 *Now soothe the whole leg by gliding your hands down one after the other.*

One hand
follows the
other

Fingertips gently
stroking

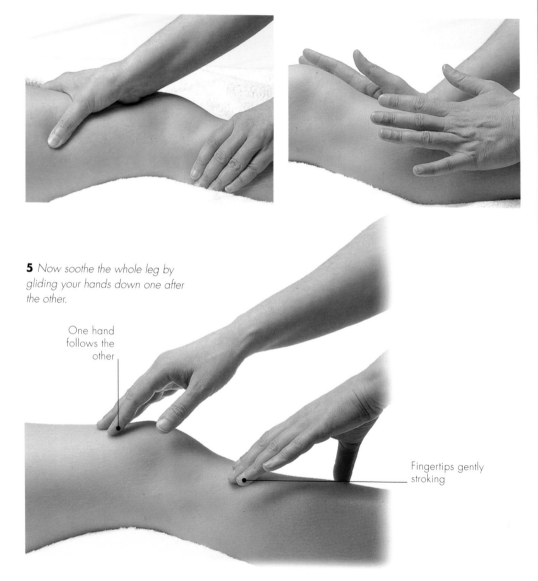

Case Study: Legs

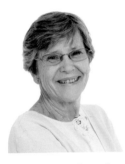

Apprehensive
Mrs. Johnson is soon put at ease about having treatment.

Consultation

Mrs. Johnson is generally fit and healthy for her age; she likes to walk as much as she can, though in the winter she sometimes finds it difficult to motivate herself. She is coming for aromatherapy to help aches in her legs and a tendency to develop swollen ankles, particularly if she hasn't been out and about very much. She lives with her daughter and their family, and sometimes feels life is rather stressful. She has never had a massage before, and is nervous about what to expect; she says she would rather the treatment concentrated on her legs.

Treatment

As her therapist, I explain to her what the treatment will entail. I reassure her that I will respect her dignity and make sure she is covered. I also agree that the first session will be best spent on the problem area, so we can try to help that and get used to each other. I look at her legs and ask her if she has seen her doctor about them. She tells me he is aware of the problem but puts it down to her age. They are a little puffy around the ankles and the feet are very pale and cold; she says her legs ache. I blend 2 drops Vetiver for the aches, 4 drops Lavender for pain relief, plus she loves the fragrance, and 4 drops Lemon to drain fluid in 4 teaspoons (20 milliliters) of carrier oil. I massage her feet and lower legs very slowly and gently, and she tells me she really enjoys it since my hands are warm. Afterward I wrap her feet up and sit them on a heatpad for a few minutes.

Self-care

Mrs. Johnson will benefit from a simple daily leg massage from her daughter for 10 minutes, using the same aromatherapy blend, and needs to raise her legs every so often during the day. A short daily walk would also be beneficial.

Timescale

It will take about five weekly 30-minute sessions to see real improvement. As Mrs. Johnson becomes more comfortable with treatment, she may even find she would like to try a full body massage, so we can really treat her holistically.

Key Essential Oil
Ginger essential oil is warming and soothing for aching muscles.

HAND MASSAGE: PALM

A hand massage is a simple and very effective treatment for a part of the body that performs many repetitive tasks each day. The movements stretch and ease out the bones and muscles. If your friend's hand is very cold, try rubbing it briskly before you begin. The hand tends to work in a closed way most of the time, and really benefits from pressure work in the palm, especially if the circulation is poor. The movements stretch out the bones and improve the circulation to the whole area. You can also give yourself a hand massage.

1 *Ask your friend to lay on their back and support the hand carefully under the wrist at all times. With the top hand, stroke from the fingers along the palm of the hand to the wrist, and glide back. Repeat four or five times.*

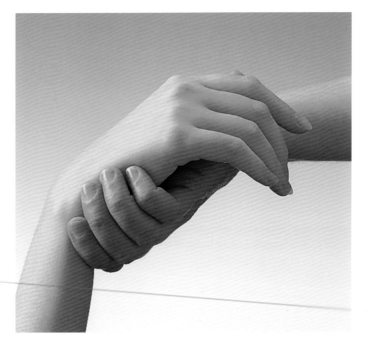

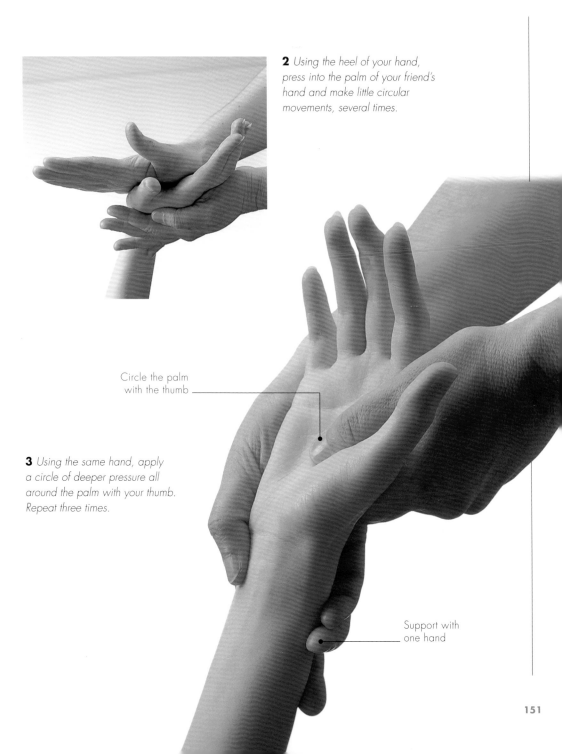

2 *Using the heel of your hand, press into the palm of your friend's hand and make little circular movements, several times.*

Circle the palm with the thumb

3 *Using the same hand, apply a circle of deeper pressure all around the palm with your thumb. Repeat three times.*

Support with one hand

151

Hand Massage: Simple Touch

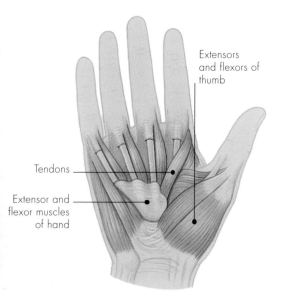

Extensors and flexors of thumb

Tendons

Extensor and flexor muscles of hand

Grasp

Muscles and ligaments allow the hand to flex and grasp.

Thousands of nerve endings in the body connect with a large proportion of the brain area, registering countless sensory messages each day. Think of all the things you touch, and how the nerves in the hand send messages to the brain. Think about how you can appreciate so many different textures, how you know without even concentrating that what you sense is alive or not. How is the bark of a tree different to plastic? Touch connects us to our feelings, too; our hands can express how we are reacting, with a clenched fist or an open palm, for example. The nerve endings make the hands incredibly sensitive to pain, heat, and cold.

Essential massage

Hand massage benefits healthy hands as well as those affected by conditions such as osteoarthritis: the circulation will improve, the skin tone may become rosy and the hand warmer. It is important to stroke very carefully and lightly if there is any injury, stiffness, or swelling in the hands. Essential oils for the circulation and muscular aches, such as Ginger, Lemongrass, and Rosemary, 3 drops each in 4 teaspoons (20 milliliters) of carrier oil, will improve movement in stiff, cold fingers.

Versatile

A hand massage is very easy to give, to anyone of any age. Because it need not involve any undressing it can be offered to people who are not used to massages in order to gain their confidence. Touching hands relieves anxiety and stress almost instantly, and is an almost instinctive response to a person in need. A hand massage works very well if you are visiting an elderly relative or someone who is ill, perhaps in a hospital; at such times it can be very helpful to have something to do that is really pleasant both to give and to receive. Touch can be magical in its effect, communicating very helpfully in circumstances where words may be difficult to find.

Key Essential Oil

Orange essential oil is sweet and pleasant to massage into the hands.

HAND MASSAGE: UPPER HAND

This concentrates a little on the fingers and the upper surface of the hand, giving a gentle stretch to the whole area. The fingers will become warm as circulation is improved. Remember to keep supporting the wrist with one hand while you work. When you have completed all the strokes on one hand, let it rest, and then repeat the whole routine on the other hand. This massage is also very easy to adapt to do to yourself.

1 *Turn the palm of the hand down. Knead and squeeze each finger in turn, followed by the thumb. Finish with a gentle pull on each one.*

2 *Apply pressure in four lines on the top of the hand from the knuckles down to the wrist, following the dips between the tendons. Don't forget the line between the thumb and first finger.*

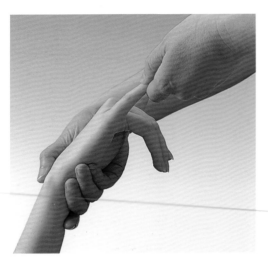

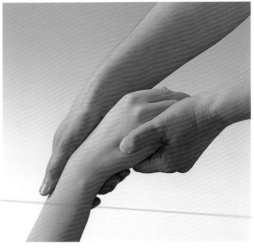

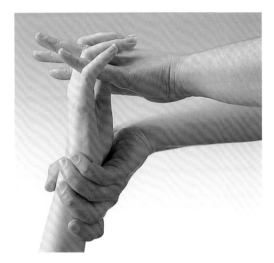

3 *Hold the wrist firmly, lace the fingers of your other hand through your friend's fingers and gently rotate the hand one way and then the other, stretching a little as you release.*

Fingers glide off

Your friend's hand is relaxed.

4 *Stroke the top of the hand from the fingers to the wrist several times, and finally, slowly glide off.*

Case Study: Hands

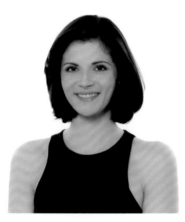

Holistic

Although Sally's problem is in her hands, she will receive a holistic treatment.

Consultation

Sally has come for some aromatherapy treatment to try to help her hands. She works as a personal assistant to a company director, and has been in her job for many years. She spends a lot of time on the computer, and her hands have begun to ache badly in the wrists, in the finger joints, and around the thumbs. She thinks she may have repetitive strain injury (RSI), where the joints have been overused in a limited way for a long period of time. She is more aware of the problem when she is stressed, which happens a lot at work. She also suffers from headaches and neck pain at the top of the shoulders. She hasn't seen her doctor about the RSI, but is having some physiotherapy to try to ease her neck.

Treatment

Massages work well alongside physiotherapy. I just suggest she lets her physiotherapist know she is coming for treatment with essential oils. Her hands do not look swollen, but they are very stiff, so I want to use painkilling and circulation-stimulating oils on them. I massage her whole body with a stress-relieving blend of Lavender, Neroli, and Frankincense, 3 drops each in 4 teaspoons (20 milliliters) of carrier oil. I then use a special blend on her hands of Lavender, Ginger, and Lemongrass, 3 drops each in 20 milliliters (4 teaspoons) of base lotion.

Self-care

Sally will massage herself using the hand blend twice a day, morning and night, between treatments. She should also have her chair position checked in relation to her computer, so that she is not straining her neck or her eyes, which may well be contributing to her headaches. Finally, she should use wrist supports or an ergonomic keyboard as she works at her computer.

Timescale

Sally will need four to six aromatherapy treatments to complement her physiotherapy. She will also benefit from gentle finger-stretching exercises and from regular self-massage to keep up the beneficial effects of the treatment she has received.

Key Essential Oil

Lemongrass essential oil is a fresh and stimulating boost to the circulation.

ARM MASSAGE: FOREARM

The arms really benefit from a massage since they are involved in most of our daytime activities. Anyone who has to lift, carry, or reach up will feel tiredness and tension in the arms at the end of a long day, which can be relieved with a massage. Try not to rush this routine; the arms need slow, careful work. Be careful to position the arm comfortably, supporting with one hand at all times.

1 *Ask your friend to lie on their back and support the arm with one hand. With the other, stroke firmly all the way up to the shoulder and glide back. Repeat four times.*

2 *With one hand supporting near the elbow, use the other hand to knead the forearm, really working the muscles between your fingers.*

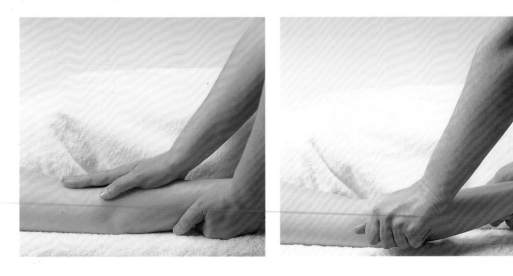

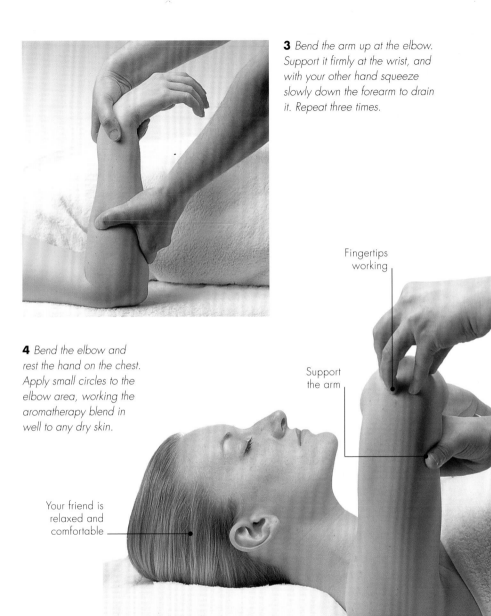

3 *Bend the arm up at the elbow. Support it firmly at the wrist, and with your other hand squeeze slowly down the forearm to drain it. Repeat three times.*

4 *Bend the elbow and rest the hand on the chest. Apply small circles to the elbow area, working the aromatherapy blend in well to any dry skin.*

Fingertips working

Support the arm

Your friend is relaxed and comfortable

159

Arm Massage for Grace & Suppleness

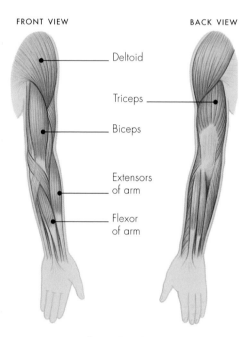

FRONT VIEW   BACK VIEW

Deltoid

Triceps

Biceps

Extensors of arm

Flexor of arm

Arm structure
The arms have amazing mobility.

You have only to watch a ballerina lift her arms above her head and pirouette to appreciate how wonderful the arms can be in motion. The anatomy of the arms is similar to the legs. The elbow allows flexibility and the muscles are arranged to allow a wide range of movement around the body. The arms may not always have muscular bulk, but they can have surprising strength as they bend, twist, lean, and curve.

Treating the arms

Aromatherapy massage is very useful for treating a range of arm-related problems, from tiredness through to muscular strain or injury. The massage needs to be combined with blends of oils that are pain-relieving, anti-inflammatory, and antispasmodic. For example, Vetiver and Sweet Marjoram are excellent oils to choose for cramping pain, and Lavender eases aches and soreness, so 3 drops each in 2 teaspoons (10 milliliters) of carrier oil is recommended for massage to local areas of pain or injury. If a muscle has been pulled, apply an ice pack first for 20 minutes, followed by a cold compress with 2 drops each Roman Chamomile and Peppermint, to relieve pain. Tennis or gardener's elbow is very common and needs oils for pain relief, such as Peppermint, Roman Chamomile,

and Lavender, 3 drops each in 2 teaspoons
(10 milliliters) of carrier oil, massaged into
the area twice a day.

Soothing massage

While self-massage can help to relieve
pain, it is also very useful to visit an
aromatherapist for the treatment of
problems in the arm; many of the key
muscles are difficult to reach yourself.
The arm massages featured here are
good if done by a partner, particularly
after activities like sports, gardening,
or lifting heavy items, when the muscles
are tight and tension can travel from the
arms to the neck region.

Key Essential Oil

Sweet Marjoram essential oil eases cramps from
aching muscles.

ARM MASSAGE: UPPER ARM

Now move to work on the upper arm, having already kneaded and drained the forearm (see pages 158–59). Some of the techniques can be adapted, depending on the muscular frame of your friend; for example, kneading can be done double- or single-handed. When you have done all the strokes on one arm, cover it, and repeat the whole routine on the other arm.

1 *Supporting the arm with one hand at the level of the elbow, stroke firmly around the shoulder in a circular movement, four or five times.*

2 *Use one hand or both to knead the upper arm, particularly the deltoid and biceps muscles. Spend a good few minutes on this.*

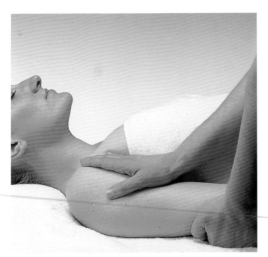

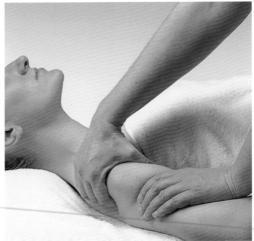

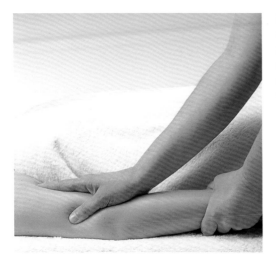

3 *Now repeat the stroke all the way up the arm from the fingers to the shoulders, but this time apply more pressure as you go up, and increase the speed to be more vigorous. This drains the whole arm.*

4 *Glide gently down the arm stroking with one hand following the other to relax the arm at the end of the massage.*

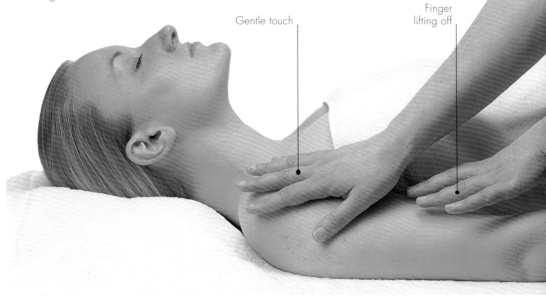

Gentle touch

Finger lifting off

The Body Language
of the Arms

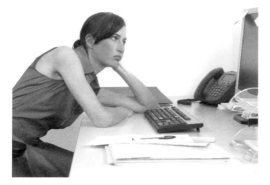

Slouch
*When concentrating on your work,
it's easy to develop bad posture.*

We may not be aware of it, but we react to surroundings and people with our arms, either wrapped around us for protection or open to meet a person on equal ground. The body language of the arms is very interesting. Notice the way people carry them, use them, and point them. The arms are very involved in what we do with our lives and the level of control we feel we may have over our circumstances.

Emotions & the body

The holistic approach to health, of which aromatherapy is a part, does not ignore the link between feelings and the body. In fact, feelings will show up in the way the body reacts to situations. It is interesting that often in a professional aromatherapy massage the arms are the most difficult part of the body to relax. They keep tensing up, going rigid, resisting the treatment. This is a sign of how much that person needs to be in control, and how much he or she needs to learn to receive. If the arms will not relax when you are working, a gentle shake of the arm should make it let go. Frequent tensing up may also indicate a lack of trust in the situation; this is why support hands are so important.

Anger, frustration, and pent-up feelings also very often rest in the arms. The tensed-up, annoyed people in that traffic jam, tapping the steering wheel or hanging onto it while cursing, may well suffer from aches in the neck and back, or even problems such as migraines, all transferred from muscles rigid with emotional frustration.

Aromatherapy in the car

The driving position we take may also contribute to aches in the neck and back. It helps to try to relax the arms as much as possible when at the wheel, not have them stretched out stiffly. It is also possible to get aromatherapy diffusers for the car. Try vaporizing a bright essential oil such as Lemon or Rosemary to improve your mood and keep you alert, and use some self-massage techniques on your shoulders while you wait. Or you can simply put drops of essential oils on a tissue and leave it on the dashboard to release its vapors into the air.

Key Essential Oil

Cypress essential oil eases aches and pains from tired muscles.

Suitable oils

*Choose warming and
soothing oils like Ginger
for abdomen massage.*

INITIAL ABDOMINAL MASSAGE

The abdomen can be a sensitive area to work on, and needs approaching with care. The solar plexus is a nerve center just below the rib cage, where we register "butterflies" in the stomach and feel fear or anxiety. Be aware of this and treat the area gently. An abdominal massage is best done calmly and smoothly, one movement flowing into another. These initial strokes are very helpful for menstrual pain, stomach cramps, or constipation.

1 *Place both hands below the navel, fingers facing upward. Stroke slowly up toward the ribs, glide out to the sides and around to the starting point. Repeat four times.*

2 *With one hand on top of the other, at your friend's right hip, stroke under the rib cage, around to the left hip, below the navel and back, in a circle. Repeat several times.*

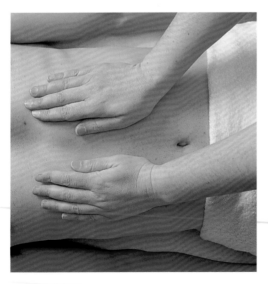

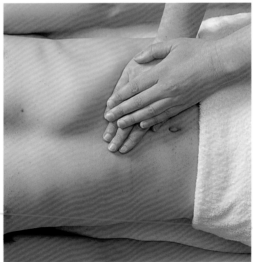

3 *Knead the abdomen from the right side to the left. Pick up the skin with care, keeping the movement firm but gentle and slow. Circle stroke a few times when you have done this.*

Be sensitive to tension

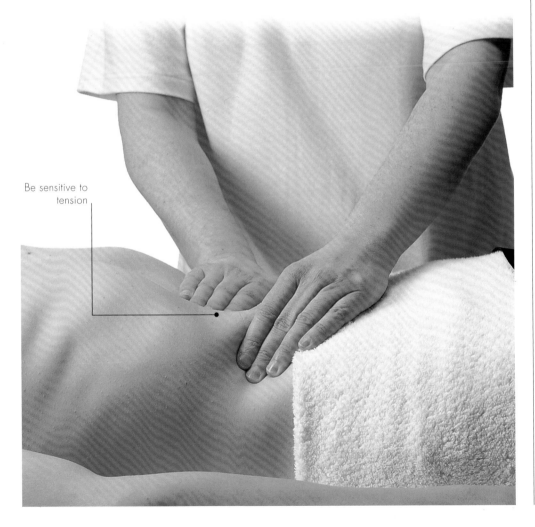

Abdominal Massage
for Digestive Problems

These muscles
flex and
rotate the
torso

Internal
and
external
oblique
muscles

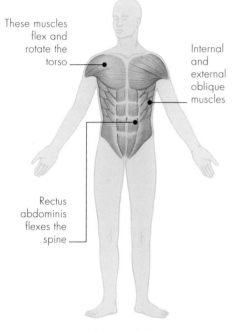

Rectus
abdominis
flexes the
spine

Inside the abdomen
*The abdominal muscles are
layered over each other.*

Digestive conditions

Common digestive problems include stomach cramps, indigestion, gas, or constipation, and in these situations massage helps to relieve pain. A circle stroke from the right to left hip can help constipation by working over the area of the large intestine, for example. Holistic aromatherapy will also consider lifestyle factors and diet in treating problems in the abdominal area.

Emotion & digestion

The digestive system is very sensitive to emotional stress, and reacts by seizing up, quite literally, to shock and trauma. Underlying emotional anxieties are very effectively treated by using Neroli. This marvelous fragrance works beautifully on the nervous system, calming anxiety and bringing deep mental relaxation. Massaged into the abdomen, Neroli also eases stomach cramps. Use 3 drops in a teaspoonful of carrier oil massaged directly into the abdomen. It can also be very effective for treating children aged

U nder the layers of skin and muscle in the abdomen are the digestive organs, constantly breaking down food, transforming the nutrients, and eliminating the waste products. We rarely notice this process unless pain indicates something is wrong.

between three and ten. In this case use
1 drop in a teaspoonful of carrier oil.
Treatment is best performed at night,
to allow the organs to rest, relax, and
release in the morning.

Digestive tonics

If the digestion is sluggish, perhaps
with constipation and diarrhea, then
digestive tonic essential oils are best used
for massage. Try 2 drops Peppermint,
2 drops Lemongrass, and 4 drops Ginger
in 3 teaspoons (15 milliliters) of carrier
oil, as a useful blend to work into the
abdomen. Massage the abdomen twice a
day and concentrate on a soothing circular
stroke. A hot water bottle over the area
is a good idea when you have finished
because the warmth is comforting.

Key Essential Oil

Ginger essential oil eases stomach cramps and
has a warming effect.

ABDOMINAL MASSAGE: TONING

Continuing to work on the whole of the abdominal region, these strokes bring a rhythmical movement to the area, gently toning all the organs. Keep to a smooth steady flow, and let the strokes have continuity with each other. Done well, an abdominal massage can be one of the most nurturing and relaxing routines to receive. Letting go of tension during a toning abdominal massage is wonderfully restful to the body and the emotions and is often the point in the massage where your friend falls asleep.

1 *Working across the area from one side to the other, let your hands trace a figure-eight shape, several times. This is a wonderful, warming stroke.*

2 *For a deeper sensation, crisscross the hands over the whole area, really lifting the muscles between your arms and hands as you work.*

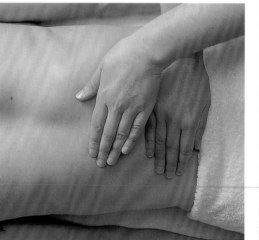
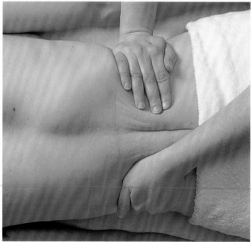

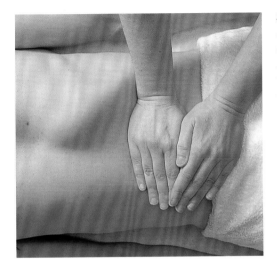

3 *Place both hands over the navel. Keep them in place and rock the area gently and slowly from side to side, pressing down alternately with your fingers and then the heels of your hands.*

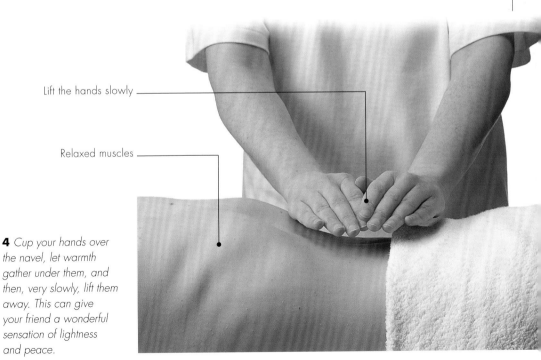

Lift the hands slowly

Relaxed muscles

4 *Cup your hands over the navel, let warmth gather under them, and then, very slowly, lift them away. This can give your friend a wonderful sensation of lightness and peace.*

171

Massage for Menstruation, Pregnancy & Labor

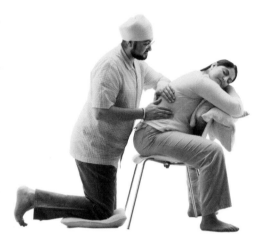

Gentle relief
Adapting a back massage like this helps in pregnancy.

Menstruation

Abdominal massage techniques are very useful for treating pain and discomfort during menstruation. They can also be self-applied quite easily (see pages 202–5). A warm bath with essential oils such as 3 drops each of Lavender and Sweet Marjoram is useful to begin with. Soak for at least 20 minutes. Then apply a blend of Lavender, Sweet

Marjoram, and Clary Sage, 3 drops each in 4 teaspoons (20 milliliters) of carrier oil, to the whole area. Remember that the pressure points around the lower back are also very effective. Finish by holding a hot water bottle wrapped in a towel over the area, and let yourself relax.

Pregnancy

There are different views about massage during pregnancy. Indigenous peoples in Africa value massages throughout pregnancy and labor. It is important to stress, however, that deep massage over the abdomen should not be carried out at this time. Gentle techniques, such as the circle stroke and the figure-eight, are very soothing, particularly in the later stages: circling over the lower back is a help for aches and pains. A soft blend for stress relief and improved rest from month three onward is 2 drops Palmarosa and 2 drops Neroli in 4 teaspoons (20 milliliters) of sweet almond oil. This is a very mild blend. For pregnancy safety advice, see page 20.

Labor

In early labor, a back massage can be very welcome, with your partner lying on her side, well-supported by pillows. Concentrate on circle stroking the lower back and the buttocks with the heel of your hand. Gentle circles can also be given over the abdomen. Between contractions, gentle strokes to the face will be calming, and the heel of the hand can also be used to massage under both feet. A blend of 2 drops Clary Sage and 2 drops Jasmine in 4 teaspoons (20 milliliters) of carrier oil can be used at that time.

Key Essential Oil

Neroli soothes and calms emotional anxiety centered in the abdomen.

NECK & SHOULDER MASSAGE • 1

The neck and shoulder area is one of the most satisfying to treat with a massage since these parts of the body immediately respond to the strokes. So much tension is stored here, and many other problems can arise if pain and immobility are not dealt with. The strokes here should feel very smooth and flowing; you are warming the area to prepare for some deeper work and you can build up a steady rhythm.

1 *Lay the friend on his back. Lean down and stretch your friend's shoulders away from the ears, pushing them gently.*

2 *Glide your hands out to the side, then draw your fingers gently back behind the shoulders and up the back of the neck. On the neck your fingers should sit on either side of the bones of the spine. Repeat four times.*

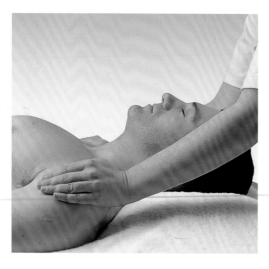

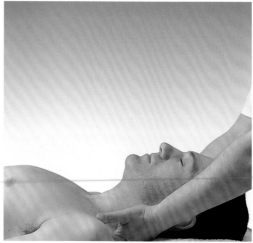

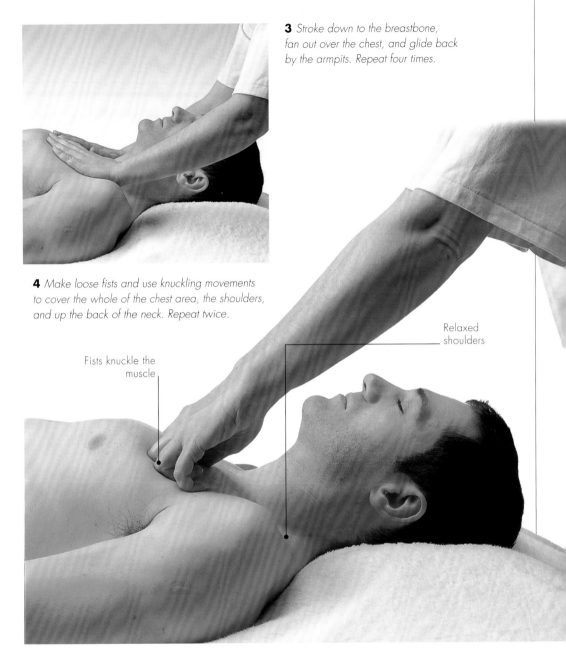

3 *Stroke down to the breastbone, fan out over the chest, and glide back by the armpits. Repeat four times.*

4 *Make loose fists and use knuckling movements to cover the whole of the chest area, the shoulders, and up the back of the neck. Repeat twice.*

Relaxed shoulders

Fists knuckle the muscle

Chronic Tension in the Neck & Shoulders

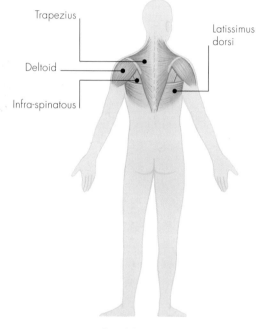

Trapezius

Latissimus dorsi

Deltoid

Infra-spinatous

Shoulder muscles

These muscles are common tension sites.

We are often totally unaware of how we sit, stand, and move around. At school, many children sit at desks that are totally unsuited to their height, and as adults, poor sitting habits continue into the office environment. So often the computer is responsible for chronic neck and shoulder tension. The head is peering up at the wrong angle, the eyes are too close, the keyboard is at the wrong height. Neck pain, eyestrain, migraines, and headaches can all result.

Everyday considerations

Simple adjustments to office furniture can radically improve day-to-day problems. Sometimes when people come for aromatherapy treatment they are surprised when the problems return after they have had some relief. If the underlying causes have not been addressed, then this is to be expected. If you sit with the phone tucked under your chin while typing with one hand, and then wonder why your neck hurts, something needs to change. The neck and shoulders are complex areas, where large muscle masses are attached to the shoulder joints and the vertebrae in the neck and the base of the skull. Too much crouching forward will overstretch the back muscles and foreshorten the chest muscles, causing stooping and excess curvature of the spine. In aromatherapy treatments, these areas are massaged and essential oils used to relieve spasm and pain. A lifestyle suggestion might be to take up yoga or t'ai chi, to rebalance the spine in the long term.

Essential treatment

Self-treatment of the area is only possible in a limited way; a partner or a professional therapist really needs to work the muscles to bring true relief. Blends such as 4 drops Rosemary, 3 drops Black Pepper, and 3 drops Vetiver in 4 teaspoons (20 milliliters) of carrier oil are very useful. The oils improve the circulation and help loosen the muscles.

Key Essential Oil

Rosemary oil increases local circulation, eases stiffness, and can also help aid muscular aches.

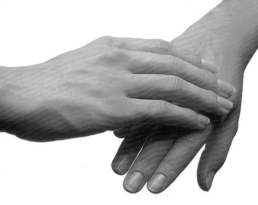

Suppleness
*Make sure you have enough
blend on your hands.*

NECK & SHOULDER MASSAGE • 2

The massage now moves a little more deeply into the neck area itself, and when you do this it is very important to feel for the neck vertebrae, keeping your fingers on either side of them. The movements are tiny, yet immensely relaxing to receive. When you have finished the routine, cover the shoulders and rest your hands over your friend's eyes for a few moments.

1 *With both hands at the base of the neck, make tiny circles all the way up either side of the neck vertebrae and glide back down. Repeat three times. At the end of the third repetition work your circles into the area immediately behind the ears.*

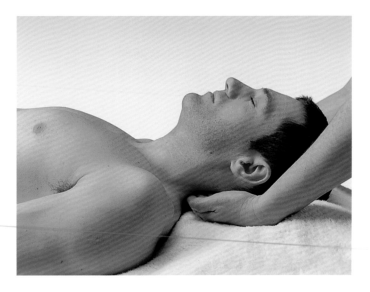

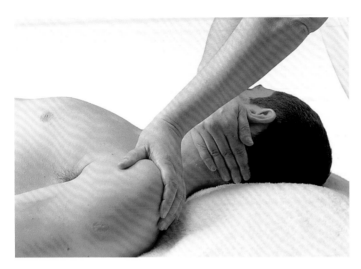

2 *Turn your friend's head comfortably to one side, and stroke up the neck, one hand quickly following the other, up to the hairline. This technique is called the Thousand Hands' Stroke. Repeat twice. Position the head gently to the other side and repeat the whole process on the other side.*

3 *Bring the head back to the center, stroke down to the breastbone, out to the shoulders, and glide off up the back of the neck. Do this three times, slowing down to finish.*

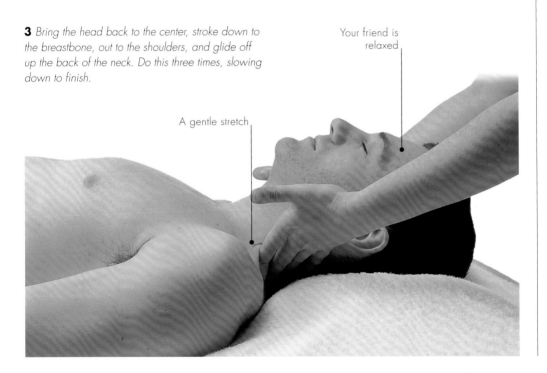

Your friend is relaxed

A gentle stretch

Case Study: Shoulder Injury

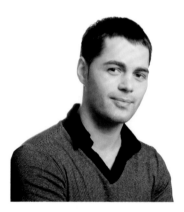

Tension
Mick is a squash enthusiast.

Consultation

Mick has come for treatment because he has pulled a muscle in his shoulder following a game of squash. He can't move very well and is in considerable pain. His girlfriend has put an ice pack on the shoulder, which has helped a little, but he feels it needs more work. The situation is made worse by the fact that he spends a lot of time driving as part of his job, and it feels worse after being in the car today. When asked about his exercise routine, he said he does not usually do any stretches or warm-ups, and on the day of the injury he was late for the game so he was in a hurry.

Treatment

It is too uncomfortable for Mick to lie face down on the couch or the floor, so I adapt the back, neck, and shoulder massage by arranging pillows on the treatment couch, sitting him on a stool, and allowing him to lean forward comfortably, supporting his arms on the couch, allowing good access to the injured area. I can treat the back, neck, and shoulders in a standing or kneeling position. I blend 3 drops Vetiver, 4 drops Sweet Marjoram, and 3 drops Peppermint in 2 teaspoons (10 milliliters) of carrier oil—a strong blend—for local application to the shoulder area and into the neck and back. I work first to warm the whole area and ease general stiffness using long strokes, followed by extensive kneading over the shoulders, specifically the injured area. I apply careful pressure around the shoulder blades, and knead again to improve local blood supply. Mick says he can feel the whole area tingling as I work.

Self-care

Once the injury improves, Mick needs to start a program of gentler exercises to warm up before his squash games. I suggest he asks fitness advisors at his gym to put together a routine. I also suggest a daily evening bath with 4 drops Lavender, 2 drops Vetiver for pain relief.

Timescale

Mick's injury could take one or two weeks to heal. He will need around four sessions from me.

Key Essential Oil

Vetiver essential oil warms and soothes deeply aching muscles.

181

FACIAL MASSAGE: UPPER FACE

A good facial massage is one of the most relaxing things to receive. The tiny little movements, if done slowly and precisely, are a real contrast to the body massage strokes, and bring a deep sense of tranquility. Make sure you wash your hands and have well-trimmed nails before you begin.

Working around the eye socket helps to tone the eyes and ease headaches or eyestrain. If you are using a blend of essential oils on the face, do keep it clear of the inner eye area, to avoid irritation.

1 *Starting with the fingers on the forehead, sweep gently down, around the temples, and over the cheeks to the chin. Then glide softly back. Repeat at least four times.*

2 *Using your thumbs or your fingertips, starting with them together in the middle of the forehead at the hairline, trace lines of very gentle pressures out to the temples, and glide back to the middle. Move a little lower and repeat, until you reach the eyebrows.*

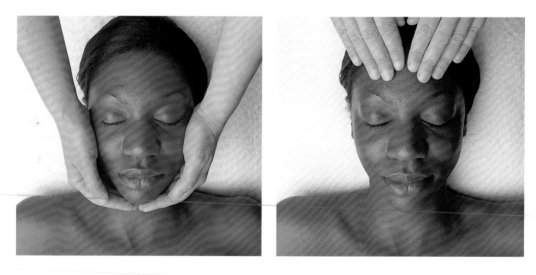

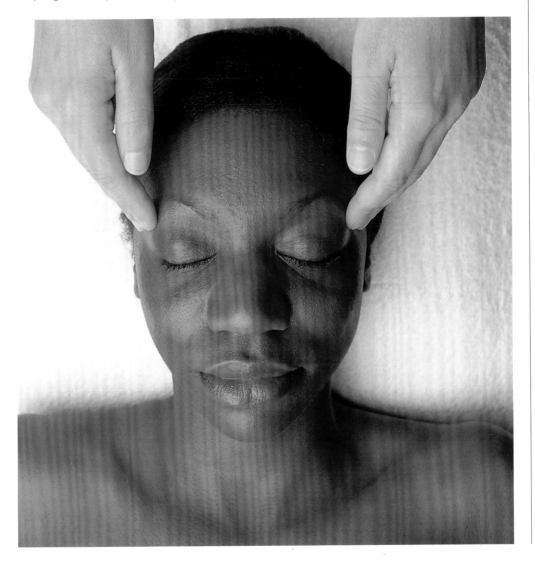

3 Now, using the tips of your middle fingers, apply a circle of tiny pressures around the bony eye socket, around under the eye, and back up the bridge of the nose. Repeat three times. Be careful to stay on the bony ridge. Do not press into the eye area itself.

The Map of the Face: Your Own Story

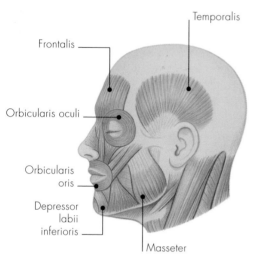

Temporalis

Frontalis

Orbicularis oculi

Orbicularis oris

Depressor labii inferioris

Masseter

Flexibility
These muscles allow a wide range of facial expression.

Every face tells a tale. The features of a Buddhist monk, deep in meditation, may be old and young at the same time. The scowl of a businessman whose train has been canceled yet again etches lines of stress across his forehead. Look at any picture of Mother Teresa, and see beyond the marks of a long life to her eyes, which looked upon suffering and coped with it. The smooth brow of a child, the clear gaze and the wide smile tell of a world as yet unexperienced, a source of wonder.

Release in relaxation

When the face is at rest, lines smooth away, the jaw loosens, the eyes close, the bones themselves seem to let go. In our waking state, we clench our teeth in frustration, narrow our gaze, and crease our foreheads in concentration. To feel someone's face release under your hands is quite an experience; you may be surprised at how much tension can be held there. The area of the jaw is a particularly common place for stiffness and even pain; grinding the teeth at night may be another sign of anxiety, and can cause headaches.

The effects of a face massage

A face massage is something of an art, and also requires patience, control of the fingers, and attention to detail. You are traveling over a map of that person, touching the face that is presented to the world, so your movements need sensitivity and care. You will soon notice how the skin warms to your touch, how the forehead releases, how the mouth relaxes. Lines seem to disappear—not permanently, but at least for a while. Give attention to the cheeks and feel the jaw let go. This massage is also very good given to those who are ill or in pain. Its gentle strokes are some of the most nurturing; along with hand massage it is a very helpful skill to offer to someone in need.

A simple face massage requires 1 teaspoon (5 milliliters) of carrier oil, together with one drop of a beautiful oil such as Rose, Neroli, or Sandalwood, for deep relaxation.

Key Essential Oil

Frankincense essential oil tones and smooths the complexion.

FACIAL MASSAGE: LOWER FACE

Now move down the face to work on the areas of the cheeks, jaw, and chin. Let the movements be slow, careful, and precise. Really concentrate on the feeling of the skin and muscles sitting over the bones of the face.

Repeat the long sweeping stroke from the very beginning (see page 182), from the forehead down the cheeks to the chin and back, three times. Then do a few slow, alternate strokes of the hands up the forehead to finish.

1 *Starting with both hands on either side of the nostrils, make tiny circles down the cheeks and jaw. Glide back and repeat at least four times.*

2 *Feel the hinge joint that opens and shuts the jaw; ask your friend to open her mouth so that you can find it. Then apply little circles to the area over that joint.*

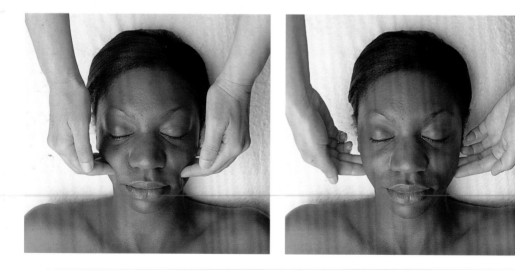

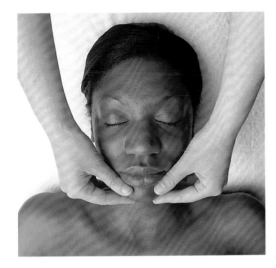

3 Bring the fingers down and knead all the way along the chin with tiny strokes, meeting in the middle. Glide back up and repeat the process at least three times.

4 Stroke the fingers alternately up the neck to the chin, sweeping them up and out. This feels really relaxing.

Facial Luxury:
Massage for the Complexion

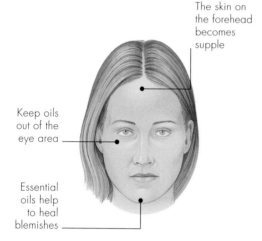

The skin on the forehead becomes supple

Keep oils out of the eye area

Essential oils help to heal blemishes

Taking time
A face massage is a nourishing beauty routine.

I t is astonishing how much money people are prepared to spend on expensive face creams, and then allow no more than a few seconds to apply it and expect it to work miracles. A good five-minute face massage each day will do as much, if not more good than these creams, especially if a blend is used containing skin-conditioning essential oils. The time you take is as important as what you use.

Essential facial oils

The flower oils are particularly good for facial work. Rose, Neroli, Ylang Ylang, Geranium, or Jasmine all nourish the skin, improving its tone and bringing a peachy glow to the complexion. If combinations are made with other skin tonic oils, such as Patchouli, Sandalwood, or Frankincense, then blemishes can be cleared and the pores tightened. Facial blends should smell wonderful.

Skin type

Before you begin, it is important to identify the skin type you will be working on. This enables you to choose the right carrier products and oils.

Dry skin is usually dull, flaking, easily chapped, tight after cleansing, and easily dehydrated. One suggestion is to use a blend of 2 drops Rose, 6 drops Sandalwood, and 2 drops Neroli in 3 teaspoons (15 milliliters) of sweet almond oil enriched with 1 teaspoon (5 milliliters) of evening primrose oil.

Oily skin is shiny and greasy, has large open pores and a coarse texture, and is prone to blackheads or acne. Try using a blend of 2 drops Ylang Ylang, 4 drops Lemon, and 4 drops Patchouli in 4 teaspoons (20 milliliters) of grapeseed oil.

Skin that is soft, supple, velvety, clear, and fine grained is known as normal. A suggested blend uses 3 drops Rose, 4 drops Frankincense, and 3 drops Neroli in 2 teaspoons (10 milliliters) of apricot kernel oil and 2 teaspoons (10 milliliters) of jojoba oil.

A dry cheek area and an oily zone down the middle of the face indicates combination skin. Use 3 drops Geranium, 4 drops Lavender, and 3 drops Orange in 4 teaspoons (20 milliliters) of jojoba oil.

Key Essential Oil

Sandalwood essential oil is an excellent all-round skin tonic.

FACIAL

The facial massage technique outlined here is based on the shiatsu pressure points and is designed to promote healthy skin as well as easing aches and pains in the face. This method can also influence other parts of the body, because the pressure points are on the meridians or energy pathways that connect the whole of the body, including the face. So a point worked on the face may well assist a separate organ that is on the same pathway.

Following the points

Following the correct sequence of points is important, and must be worked on both the left and right sides. Use one of your fingers or your thumb, and hold each point for around 5 seconds, in a way that is noticeable but not over-painful. Make sure your nails are trimmed short.

Working in order

Follow the sequence on the right to achieve the best results.

The Pressure Points

Point 1 Trace a line from the middle of the eyebrows back to the middle of the head, press once here.

Point 2 Press the temples at the hairline on each side.

Point 3 Press approximately $3/8$ inch (1 centimeter) away from the corner of the eye, on either side.

Point 4 Press once between the eyebrows.

Point 5 Press carefully on both sides, deep in the corner of the eye.

Point 6 Press on both sides directly under the pupil, on the border of the cheekbone.

Point 7 Press on both sides, two finger widths below point 6.

Point 8 Press on both sides at the corners of the mouth, below point 7.

Point 9 Press on both sides next to the nostrils.

Point 10 Ask your friend to tense the jaw and you will find a small hollow with your fingers. Ask your friend to relax the jaw and press on both sides.

Point 11 Press carefully on either side of the voicebox in the throat.

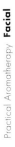

The pressure points

Facial massage
techniques are based
on the ancient principles
of the shiatsu system.

Pressure Points & the Complexion

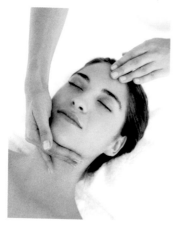

Wide-ranging uses
*Points on the face can help soothe
other parts of the body.*

It is good to incorporate the pressure points into a facial care program for extra attention to the complexion, two or three times a week. Try working the sequence before you do any massage with an essential oil blend, because your fingers are working close to the eyes, and essential oils are best kept out of the delicate eye area. Once you have completed the points, then apply your blend.

Links to other areas

The facial pressure points have some useful links to other problems, as well as helping to improve the complexion overall. Point 1 helps to stimulate hair growth and soothes headaches and stress. Point 2 soothes headaches and tired eyes. Point 3 is also good for headaches and eye problems. Point 4 helps sinusitis and a blocked nose, as well as tension. Point 5 helps concentration, inner focus, and tired eyes. Point 6 helps blocked passages, sinus pain, and digestive problems. Point 7 relieves facial tension. Point 8 helps stomach cramps and facial tension. Point 9 relieves congestion and colds. Point 10 helps ease tension in the jaw and is also good for migraines. Point 11 stimulates the thyroid gland and influences hormone balance. Point 11 has been used as a beautifying massage for thousands of years in India and the East and is credited in some texts with enhancing and maintaining beauty.

General stress relief

Working these points is also very good for relieving stress and tension, but remember that you need to keep the pressure gentle, so that it does not become uncomfortable. This routine can be used as self-massage, to relax the face during the daytime if you work in an office, staring at a computer screen, for example, because it takes only a few minutes to do.

Points 2, 3, and 4 can also be worked with one drop of neat Lavender oil, keeping well away from the inner eye area, if you feel the threat of a headache or migraine.

If you grind your teeth at night or suffer from migraines, try massaging point 10 with a drop of Lavender before you sleep.

Key Essential Oil

Neat **Lavender** essential oil is excellent for local pain relief.

Beneficial

Apricot kernel oil is one of the most useful for normal skins.

SELF-TREATMENT FOR FACIAL CARE Essential oils,

aromatherapy blends, and simple massages can become a pleasant natural beauty routine, which is absolutely free of chemicals and artificial ingredients. As you incorporate these elements into your life—in the form of face masks, toners, and creams or lotions—you will also experience the destressing quality of aromatherapy.

1 *In a small dish place 2 tablespoons (30 milliliters) of organic live yogurt.*

2 *Add 1 teaspoon (5 milliliters) of jojoba oil and stir in.*

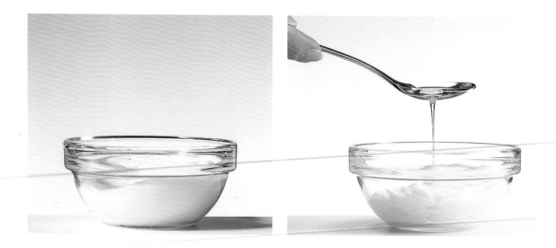

Daytime

In the morning, apply essential oils in either a cream or a lotion base, which will not leave an oily residue. First cleanse the face; next use a flower water toner on it; and then apply your cream or lotion blend to prepare the skin for make-up.

Night-time

When you apply blends to your face in the evening, they are absorbed into the skin while you sleep. Cleanse the face, tone with a flower water, and apply a cream or facial oil using the face massage techniques described on pages 182–87.

3 *Add a total of 3 drops essential oil to the mixture. A simple blend would be 1 drop Geranium and 2 drops Frankincense. Stir in.*

Yogurt Face Mask

As a weekly treat, make up this special face mask. The yogurt nourishes the skin and the jojoba oil provides a conditioning treatment, as well as dispersing the essential oils.

4 *Apply the mask to the skin. Leave for 15 minutes. Remove with a cotton ball soaked in warm water, then tone the skin with rose water. Let the skin breathe for an hour before applying any cream.*

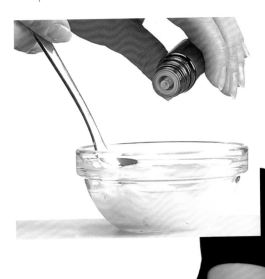

Aromatherapy Facial Care Preparations

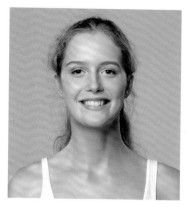

Skincare

Use aromatherapy blends to enhance your complexion.

It is possible to make simple facial preparations at home. If you prefer to buy your base products, check that moisturizing creams are free of animal-derived or petroleum-based elements. Good essential oil blends are: for dry, normal, or mature skin, 3 drops Geranium, 4 drops Sandalwood, 3 drops Orange; for oily or blemished skin, 3 drops Frankincense, 4 drops Lavender, 3 drops Juniper; and for sensitive skin, 2 drops Palmarosa and 3 drops Roman Chamomile.

Moisturizer

Makes about 12 teaspoons (60 grams)

4 teaspoons (20 grams) beeswax
4 teaspoons (20 milliliters) sweet almond oil
4 teaspoons (20 milliliters) rose water

You will also need a deep-sided pot, a heat-resistant glass dish to sit over the pot like a double boiler, and a 2-ounce (60-gram) amber glass jar, available from a pharmacy.

Heat the beeswax and sweet almond oil together in a glass dish over a pot of simmering water until the wax melts. Keep stirring and add the rosewater to the mixture drop by drop until it is all absorbed. Remove from the heat and stir until the mixture cools. Add up to 10 drops of your chosen essential oils and stir into the mixture. Pour into the glass jar and refrigerate.

This light cream makes a good aftershave balm for men. Try adding 3 drops Patchouli, 3 drops Frankincense, and 4 drops Atlas Cedarwood essential oil.

For mature skin, try adding 3 drops Rose, 4 drops Neroli, and 3 drops Sandalwood to the cream for a beautiful, soothing blend to enhance the texture of the skin and make it peachy soft.

Toner

Essential oil suppliers and good health food
retailers are able to supply flowerwaters, called
hydrolats, which are the by-products of essential
oil distillation. Rosewater, lavender water, and
orangeflower water are all excellent to use as
facial toners. Keep in the refrigerator for up to
6 months.

Cleanser

Makes about 12 teaspoons (60 grams)

1 teaspoon (5 grams) beeswax
8 teaspoons (40 milliliters) jojoba oil
2 teaspoons (10 grams) cocoa butter

You will also need a deep-sided pot, a heat-
resistant glass dish to sit over the pot like a double
boiler, and a 2-ounce (60-gram) amber glass jar,
available from a pharmacy.

Melt the beeswax in the glass dish over a pot of
simmering water. Add the jojoba oil and cocoa
butter and stir well. Remove from the heat and stir
until the mixture cools a little. Add a total of 10
drops of chosen essential oils and stir in. Pour the
mixture into the glass jar and refrigerate it. Apply
sparingly, work into the skin and wipe off with a
cotton ball. Follow with a flowerwater toner.

ASSAGE: HANDS

It is all too easy to forget about relaxation in the busy rush of day-to-day life. Yet there are simple self-massage techniques that you can easily use on yourself without taking up much time at all. Some, like this routine for the hands and elbows, can even be done at work. You may wish to nourish your skin with a hand cream, a skin care lotion, or a carrier oil blend (see pages 100–17).

1 *Stroke the upper surface of one hand with the other hand, from the fingers to the wrist. Repeat four times.*

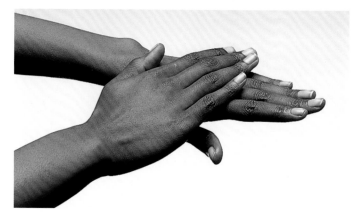

2 *Turn the palm upward. Use your other thumb to make a circle of small pressures all around the inner surface of the hand. Repeat three times.*

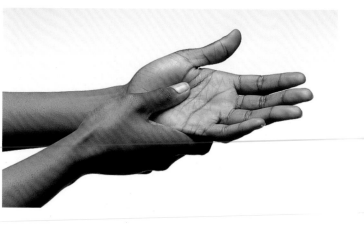

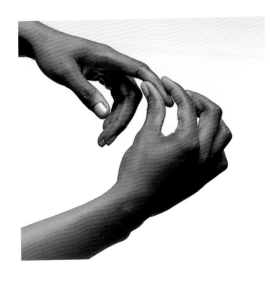

3 *Carefully massage each finger in turn, from the tip to the base and back, also working on the thumb. Repeat this stroke up and down the hand. Repeat the whole routine on the other hand.*

4 *After a bath or shower, pay special attention to the elbows, making little circular movements.*

Self-Massage:
A Caring Touch

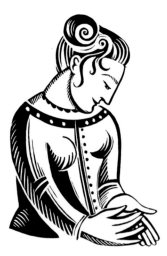

Napoleonic beauty care
The Empress Josephine used an almond oil hand cream.

The hands need special attention to take care of dry skin, to nourish the nailbed and the nails, and ease aches and pains from everyday repetitive tasks. Aromatherapy blends and massage can achieve all this very pleasantly. Once a week, try this treat for the hands, ideally in the evening after a bath or shower, since oils are better absorbed through damp skin and have time to sink in while you sleep.

The hands

Start by gently brushing the hands while they are dry, working on the fingers and the palms. Add a small glass of whole milk and 3 drops Mandarin to a bowl of warm water. Dip the hands in the water and milk and let them soak for 10 minutes. Then pat them dry.

File the nails smooth, and gently push back the cuticles. Take a blend of 3 drops Rose, 3 drops Patchouli, and 4 drops Sandalwood in 4 teaspoons (20 milliliters) of sweet almond oil, and apply to your hands using the self-massage routine described on pages 198–99. Really work the blend into the fingers, the nailbed, and the nails, and any particularly dry areas.

If your hands are particularly dry and chapped you could use jojoba oil instead of sweet almond oil, for extra conditioning. As you work, feel how good it is to give time and care to your hands, which work hard for you every day. Remember that the hand massage also helps poor circulation and stiffness, and can be repeated as often as necessary to improve mobility and suppleness.

The elbows

The elbow area is very prone to dryness, and is often ignored. A rich carrier oil such as sweet almond, jojoba, or evening primrose is well worth applying twice a day. Use one teaspoonful of oil, enriched with 1 drop Rose, Neroli, or Sandalwood. Alternatively, you could use the hand blend mentioned above for a massage of the whole arm: after the hand routine, using long sweeping strokes to work the blend in from the shoulder right down to the fingers. Then use your fingertips to really massage the elbows effectively.

Key Essential Oil

Rose is a classic soothing ingredient in a handcare cream.

SELF-MASSAGE: ABDOMEN & HIPS

The abdomen and hips really benefit from self-massage to relieve aches and pains, as well as to tone and condition the skin. It is best to do this routine in the evening, after a bath or shower, because the oils are absorbed better through damp skin and have time to sink in while you sleep.

1 *Lying comfortably on your back, with one hand on top of the other, start at the right hip. Circle under your ribs, to the left hip, and back over your lower abdomen. Repeat several times, in a steady rhythm.*

2 *Using your right hand, make a figure-eight movement across the abdomen. Repeat four times.*

3 *Pick up and knead the abdomen from the right side to the left, and back again. Repeat twice. Circle stroke a few times after this.*

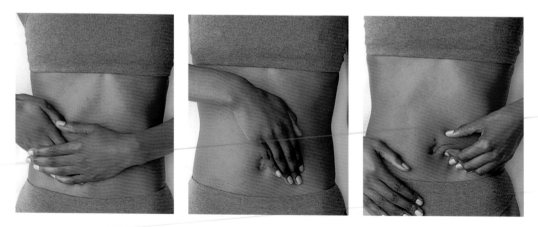

4 *Cup both hands over the navel, wait until the heat gathers, then lift off.*

5 *Roll onto your right hip and circle stroke all around your left hip several times.*

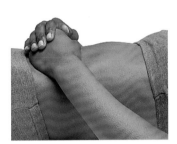

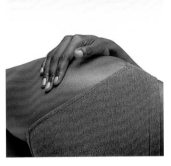

6 *Using loose fists, gently pummel the hip to stimulate the circulation. Smooth the area with more circle strokes to finish, then repeat the routine on the other side.*

Self-Massage for Relaxation & Pain Relief

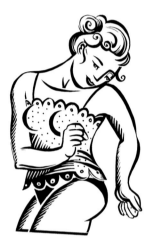

Hip massage
*Pummeling the hips improves
circulation in that area.*

Abdominal and hip massage is very beneficial for stress relief, general tension, and pain relief. It is a good idea to make sure you will not be abruptly disturbed while carrying out abdominal self-massage techniques, so that you can really make the most of the experience. Self-massage helps to relax you before sleep, so you have better-quality rest and are more likely to wake up refreshed.

Relief recipes

There are a number of specific problems that can be relieved using essential oil blends and the abdominal and hip self-massage described on pages 202–3. The circle stroke is one of the best and most comforting to do for yourself for simple pain relief, and when the oil has been applied, wrap a hot water bottle in a towel and apply it to the abdomen to help you relax.

For menstrual cramps, try a blend of 5 drops Sweet Marjoram, 3 drops Clary Sage, and 2 drops Vetiver in 4 teaspoons (20 milliliters) of grapeseed oil.

If you suffer from indigestion, constipation, or sluggish digestion use 4 drops Ginger, 2 drops Peppermint, and 4 drops Black Pepper in 4 teaspoons (20 milliliters) of sweet almond oil.

Stress-related stomach cramps can be relieved using a blend of 3 drops Neroli, 3 drops Sandalwood, and 4 drops Lavender in 4 teaspoons (20 milliliters) of grapeseed oil.

Pregnancy

If you are pregnant, just do the circle stroke on yourself, very gently. As the abdomen warms it is lovely to send nurturing thoughts to your baby. A good blend to use after the third month would be 2 drops Palmarosa and 2 drops Neroli in 4 teaspoons (20 milliliters) of sweet almond oil. For pregnancy safety advice, see page 20.

Essential hip blends

For the hip area, if you are conscious of poor skin tone, try skin-brushing first, to stimulate local circulation, then be quite vigorous about your massage. Circle strokes, pummeling, then knuckling are useful techniques, always soothing the skin with circles to finish. Use cleansing oils such as Fennel and Juniper.

Key Essential Oil

Clary Sage essential oil is gentle and soothing to menstrual cramps.

SELF-MASSAGE: THIGHS & FEET

The thighs are a popular area for self-massage; it's important to massage them regularly, as frequent work on the thighs is needed to improve the skin tone. The feet can be massaged at any time to help with poor circulation. Remember that any of the techniques for the foot massage described on pages 134–39 can also be adapted for self-massage.

1 *Sitting comfortably with one leg bent, stroke up the thigh toward the hip and glide back down to the knee. Pressure should be aimed upward, toward the hip. Repeat several times.*

2 *Pick up and knead the thigh, first on the outside and then the inside.*

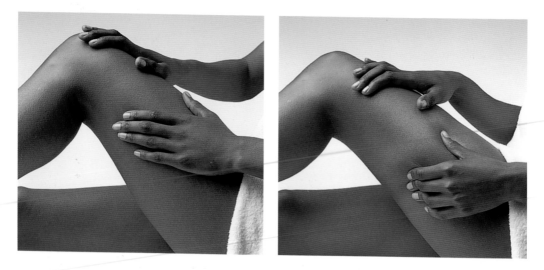

3 *With both fists held loosely, pummel the thigh area thoroughly but gently, then soothe the area with circle strokes. Repeat the whole process on the other thigh.*

4 *Sit with one foot balanced on your knee, and sandwich both your hands around it, one hand above, the other below. Stroke from the ankle to the toes and back, several times.*

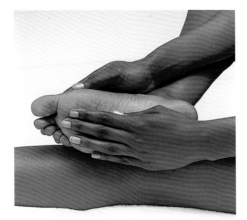

5 *Making a loose fist, knuckle all over the underside of the foot. Sandwich stroke again a few times to finish. Repeat the routine on the other foot.*

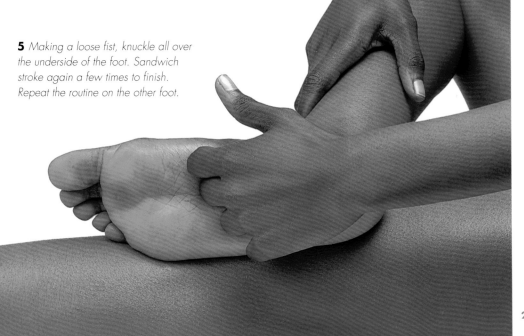

Self-Massage to Tone & Revitalize

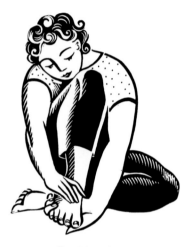

Foot treats
*After a long day it is good
to massage the feet.*

So often people ask about massages, oils, and cellulite, as if there were a miracle cure. Professional lymphatic drainage and deep tissue work are really needed to make a major difference, but self-massage can be useful, provided it is done regularly. A few minutes each day is better than an hour whenever you happen to remember. Try to incorporate techniques into your daily routine.

Basic toning

You can carry out useful toning techniques every day at home, such as skin-brushing the dry skin area before you take a shower and using alternate cool and comfortably hot jets of water in the shower over the affected area to improve circulation. Be sensible; ice cold and boiling hot are not what is meant. Follow with a firm massage (see pages 206–7) and use the leg routine described on pages 142–47, adapting the strokes for self-massage. Knuckling is very good over the thigh area.

Essential toning oils

A suitable essential oil toning blend for the thighs is 3 drops Cypress, 3 drops Rosemary, and 4 drops Lemon in 4 teaspoons (20 milliliters) of grapeseed oil. You could also spread the blend in a massage that continues down the leg to include the calf muscles as well, on the way to the feet. This blend also helps aches after playing sports.

Essential footcare oils

A foot massage is so relaxing to do for yourself at the end of a long hard day. If you have a foot spa, then start with that as a treat for the feet; if not, then soak the feet in a large bowl of warm water with a teacupful of Epsom or Dead Sea mineral salts added, along with 1 drop Peppermint and 2 drops Lavender. Soak for about 15 minutes. Dry the feet, then massage in either a carrier oil blend or a cream to help callouses and dry skin, as well as the circulation. A useful blend to try mixes 3 drops Black Pepper, 3 drops Peppermint, and 4 drops Rosemary in 4 teaspoons (20 milliliters) of carrier oil or base cream. Really work the blend well into the heels and toes, and any dry areas.

Key Essential Oil

Cypress is an excellent circulation stimulant and general tonic.

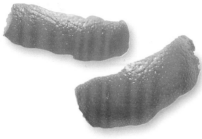

Zest for life

Orange peel added to bathwater will scent and enliven it.

ORANGE PEEL

SCENTED BATHING
Taking essential oil baths can very quickly become a well-loved part of your daily routine. It is a particularly good idea at night, as a way of destressing at the end of a long hard day. Try to create a sanctuary—even the simplest bathroom can be transformed with a few candles, some music, and warm fluffy towels to wrap yourself up in.

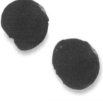

ROSE PETALS

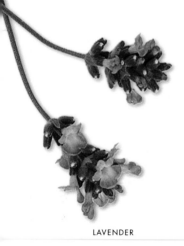

LAVENDER

Herbs & crystals

In the past, herb sachets were infused in bathwater to give a fragrance. Essential oils are much more concentrated than herbs, so just a couple of drops of your favorites will be all you need. A few rose petals, dried lavender flowers, or sprigs of herbs such as rosemary, marjoram, or peppermint can float on the water surface for added interest. Some people like to take a bath with a favorite crystal in the water; rose quartz is pleasant to try. Consider an aromatherapy bath as a treatment and allow at least 20 minutes for it. Breathe deeply and enjoy.

A milk bath

In 6 teaspoons (30 milliliters) whole milk, add 3 drops each of two favorite essential oils. Stir well, pour into the hot water, and swirl to disperse.

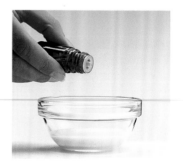

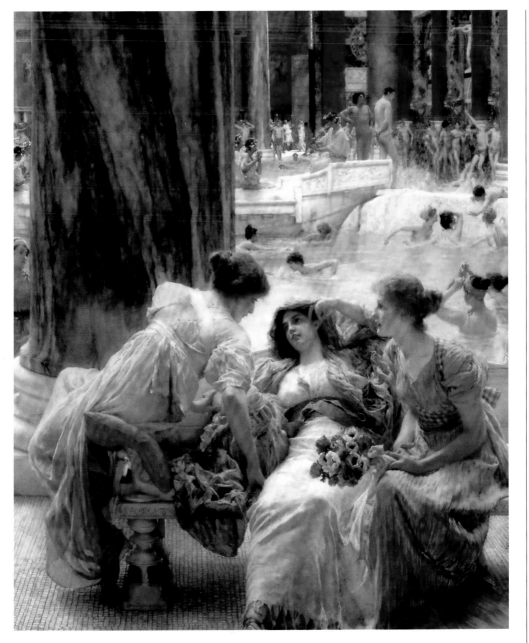

Languid beauty
Communal bathing depicted by a romantic artist of the Victorian era.

Scented Bathing: Useful Tips & Blends

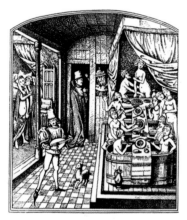

Bath time
Mass bathing in public bathhouses
was common in medieval times.

To experience a truly wonderful essential oil bath, there a few things you should remember.

Essential bathing

Always run the bath water before you add the oils. Then add your oils to the surface and swish the water gently before getting in. In total, 4–6 drops of essential oils is recommended in a bath. You can mix your oils in carrier oil if you wish, but this is not necessary, since only a few drops of oil are diluted in the bathwater, and it can be messy to clean. You can use a milk bath instead.

It is important that you really allow time to soak in the water before you use any soap, which will buffer the skin against the oils, and slow down their absorption. If possible, don't use soap at all. Use a shower to get clean first.

And finally, make sure that you use an appropriate cleaning product for enamel or plastic surfaces after your bath; some oils leave a sticky residue.

Bathe like royalty

Queen Cleopatra is said to have bathed in asses' milk for her complexion. You can recreate the same nourishing, luxurious effect by pouring 6 teaspoons (30 milliliters) of whole milk into a glass, adding your chosen essential oils and swishing the mixture into the bath. Your skin will feel lovely afterward and the experience is utterly luxurious.

Detoxify

A bath with a teacupful of Dead Sea
mineral salts will aid detoxification. Add
4 drops Lemon and 2 drops Juniper and
follow with a cellulite massage blend.

Showers

Use one of the good quality shower
gels containing essential oils which
are available on the market.

Bath Blends

Here are a few blends you might like to try for specific soothing or emotional
effects. The numbers next to the oils refer to the number of drops to be used.

Total Destress
2 Jasmine
3 Mandarin

Exotic Retreat
3 Bergamot
2 Ylang Ylang

Indian Sunset
3 Sandalwood
1 Rose
2 Patchouli

Sleepy Head
4 Lavender
2 Neroli

Breathe Deep
3 Atlas Cedarwood
2 Lemon

Cloud Nine
3 Neroli
2 Frankincense

Cleopatra
2 Rose
1 Patchouli
2 Orange

Children's Bathtime
2 Mandarin
2 Roman Chamomile

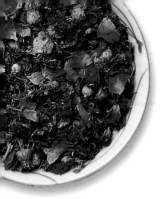

Potpourri

Bring the magic of aromatherapy into your environment.

THE HOME There is more to aromatherapy than massages and baths. There are a number of other ways you can use essential oils around your home to create a pleasant atmosphere and personalize your space with wonderful fragrances.

Pillows

Try two drops of either Lavender or Orange on the pillowcase before sleep.

Writing paper

Try scenting your correspondence with a drop of Orange, Lemon, or Mandarin.

First aid

Lavender and Tea Tree oils are a must for the first-aid box.

Disinfectant

Using 3 drops of Eucalyptus or Tea Tree is helpful in the bathroom.

Curtains & furniture

*Try 2 drops Black Pepper or
2 drops Lemon to keep cats off.*

Burners

*Essential oil burners work well in living
rooms, bedrooms, and hallways, to
personalize your space, or create a
special atmosphere. Remember to keep
an eye on flame-driven burners, or,
alternatively, there are very effective
electrical ones available.*

Room fresheners

*Try using 2 drops Peppermint or
2 drops Lemongrass on a carpet.
Leave the oils to evaporate to get
rid of smoke or pet odors.*

GLOSSARY

Analgesic pain relieving

Antibacterial controls bacterial infection

Antidepressant relieves low moods

Antifungal controls fungal infection

Anti-inflammatory reduces swelling or redness

Antispasmodic aids the easing of cramp

Antiviral stimulates the body's immune response

Base cream/lotion a carrier product that is suited to specific uses and is particularly good for the skin

Carrier oil a vegetable oil used to dilute an essential oil and make it safe for use in massage

Detoxifying assists in cleansing the system

Digestive tonic improves the digestive function

Distillation the extraction of essential oils by steam pressure and condensation

Diuretic increases urinary flow

Essential oil a concentrated, fragrant oil that is extracted from the leaves, flowers, twigs, fruit, or roots of a plant

Expectorant expels mucus from the respiratory tract

Expression the extraction of essential oils by pressing the peel of fruit (especially citrus fruit)

Fragrance notes the classification of a fragance in terms of top, middle, and base notes, depending on its intensity and how quickly it evaporates

Genito-urinary tonic improves the function of the bladder and sexual organs

Hypertensive increases blood pressure

Hypotensive lowers blood pressure

Immune tonic improves the body's natural defenses

Local circulation stimulant reddens and warms the skin

Menstrual regulator brings the monthly cycles into balance

Patch test a test of an essential oil on the inside of the wrist or elbow crease to establish whether any adverse reaction will occur

Phototoxic may cause irregular patches on skin in UV light

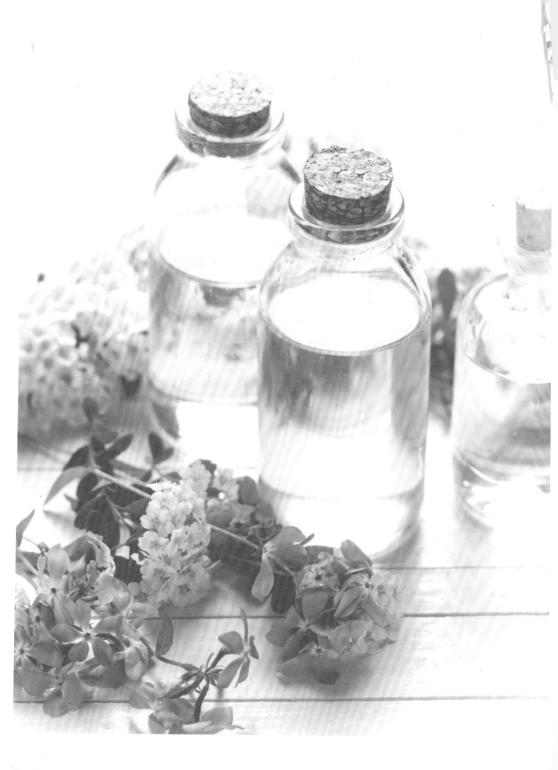

SECRETS OF
AROMATHERAPY